The Diabetes Decoder

Recognize and Reprogram
Your Diabetes Myths

The Diabetes Decoder

Recognize and Reprogram
Your Diabetes Myths

Sheri Fawson

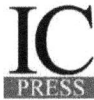

IC
PRESS

Idea Creations Press
www.ideacreationspress.com

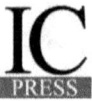

IC Idea Creations Press
www.ideacreationspress.com

The methods discussed here are stress management techniques that are easily and quickly mastered by many people. They are not intended to take the place of psychotherapy. People who have medical or emotional problems that require professional attention should use these programs as they would any other stress relief method, and under the supervision of a physician or other qualified health professional.

Library of Congress Control Number: 2016946581

ISBN-13: 9780996665773
ISBN-10: 0996665773

Printed in the U.S.A.

For my mom who didn't know if I would make it

"Have you ever seen a case of seasickness this bad?" I asked him.

"No. Not this bad. I think it's something else, making it worse," he said. "There are a few things we could do. We could try to radio for a boat to take you to the main island, or we could take you ashore in the dingy. There are some lounge chairs on the beach. You could sleep on them until morning and then decide what to do." Since it was three a.m. we decided on that option and he took us ashore.

Soon after the captain went back to the boat we realized our error. We should have brought my insulin. I had not brought a glucometer on the trip, the device to test my blood sugar, but by now I knew it was really high. On the boat I had not thought about it: I had not been able to think.

Glade hadn't thought about insulin either. He had never had to think about it in nearly eight years since I had developed diabetes. He said, "I love you, but I don't know what to do."

Acknowledgments

This book has been the culmination of more than 30 years of searching for answers to my many, many questions. Thank you to all who contributed. First a huge thanks to my husband Glade and my wonderful adult children Ty and Chelsea, for your patience, your encouragement, and all the love I need in this world. You bore the brunt of my sickness and frustration and yet you hung in there until I could become the person I am really meant to be. I don't know why – may be you thought you had to. But I appreciate it.

Thanks to all my mentors, and especially to David Butler, my first coach, Jack Canfield, who is definitely the world's finest coach, and Wade Lindstrom of PEI, who saw greatness in me before I could see it. And to the many people I have coached, I hope this book finds its way into your hands. You have taught me more than anyone about resilience and what it takes to power through difficulties and come out shining. You continue to inspire me and I hope I can live up to your expectations. It would be great to reconnect with you.

Thanks Mom and Dad for the good and the bad. I am sorry for the bad I caused and hope you can be proud of me for who I have become through it all. And Carol, Barbara, Diane, Ann, and Bruce, my five sweet siblings, thank you for being there, for your patience, and for listening to me. I thank you all especially for those many years ago when what I asked for was your understanding and you did much more; you joined me in my decision to confront. Ann, many of our long conversations found their way onto these pages and I thank you for them.

My editors Kathryn and Doug Jones waited for me for what seemed like forever to finally help me get published and your input and wisdom have been invaluable. I honestly did not know where to go to get this done. Thank you for staying on board while I sorted through the hardest part of publishing, the waiting. The result is worth it and I am happy to have had the honor of your guidance.

Thank you, future readers and I hope you find what you need here. It has been a privilege.

Sheri Fawson

Contents

Introduction

Experts have written plenty of books on the physical aspects of managing diabetes. I recommend many of them and have listed my favorites in the back; however, we'll be taking a very different approach. Most people who have diabetes aren't happy with their lives, yet we tend to believe this is as good as it's ever going to get. I listened to that argument in my own head for a long time; the more I listened the longer it took to get started changing my paradigm. To understand my unique approach you must first acknowledge that inside every disease is a message. There is a purpose to your circumstances and a deeper meaning than there appears to be at first glance. If you begin to sort through the mental, emotional, social, and spiritual elements of your life you can change your internal environment from toxic to healthy in every way, resulting in an easier life that is fuller than you could have imagined.

All my health care professionals could not have created a philosophy and developed the right code for me. I was the only one who could do that and due to my extreme unhappiness, little by little through blood testing, sweat, and tears, I did it. I did not see it for the longest time, despite how simple it was. But once I understood, once I realized I had the ability to create a life I wanted instead, my second major breakthrough, the solution to making it easy, showed up.

Everywhere people who have diabetes feel exhausted from the mess of having to take care of it. They feel guilty about the energy drain on their tired loved ones, sad about their lost health, ashamed of their failures, and frustrated about lost hopes and dreams. We are fragile and we tend to readily give up. After all, for those of us with Type 1, our islet cells didn't survive the toxic environment of our own bodies. Our world, the foods we eat, and our very lives are toxic environments too, and many with diabetes are merely surviving it – not really living.

But if your *mess* is your *mess*-age, what can be learned? The mind does funny things; it will tell you you're not special. My mind played a constant looped recording that said I had nothing special to give to anyone. Yet I know there are ways to heal from our disease – much more than watching our carb intake and all the other things people with diabetes must do. Healing does not necessarily mean you no longer need to take insulin or count your carbohydrates. For many of us there is no known "cure," but there is freedom from being held hostage by our own feelings. Within your most profound experiences lies the essence of what will be your greatest contribution to humankind. And you can make that contribution once you have begun to heal.

You will bring an end to the drama when you start making choices that will give you the best possible life, and help you create your very best version of you. But it will be important to work through your grief, guilt, anger, sorrow, and fear to become happy about it. Happy, not in spite of having diabetes but happy *with* it – accepting an experience that is very much a part of who you are, and yet does not define you.

Why would you choose to endure pain? Why would you remain helpless while watching someone you love choose to endure it? In this manual I propose powerful solutions to help you stop merely enduring and start really living. This book is for you if you feel these words ringing true.

There's more to diabetes management than understanding food, watching carbohydrates, monitoring blood sugar, and getting enough exercise. You also need a good road map. Your doctor tells you everything you need to know, right?

Introduction

Don't get me wrong, everyone who has diabetes needs health care providers. Rule number one is talking with your doctor. Your doctor will do his job, which is to teach you to survive the disease by monitoring your blood sugar and maintaining tight control of your glucose levels. Most likely your doctor won't teach you how to test when you don't feel like it. And he probably won't teach you how to *thrive* in the toxic environment of diabetes, or how to develop a philosophy that actually helps you do it. For one, he assumes you'll figure that part out. Plus, it's not his job.

From a logical perspective life is almost never fair. And feeling it is unfair hinders good diabetes self-care. There are ways you can protect yourself from some events and elements, and we will discuss those strategies, but in every life rain must fall. You will need another perspective to begin to look at diabetes not as a typhoon but as a rain shower.

The techniques within this book are simple enough; it's learning to embrace adversity that's not as easy. To cut through the myriad reasons that are stopping you will require commitment. To begin with, as best you can, try to not resist the things you dread. As best you can, start to take a more critical look at the beliefs, attitudes, and behaviors that keep your life DIS-eased* and insignificant. That's the first step toward creating your authentic code.

No one-size-fits-all routine can make you a happy person with diabetes. A system that is ideal for one person may be entirely wrong for another. Just continue solving until you hit on the right combination of elements – like opening a safe. We will discuss the structure of your unique code in detail but I wish to add that your structure must include practices that sustain your spiritual well-being.

Your spirituality is vital for creating the ideal conditions needed

---

*The term DIS-ease refers to the idea that *disease* and being ill-at-ease or *dis-eased* are synonymous, a point made throughout the book.

to thrive in your body's toxic environment, as well as to create within you a *nontoxic* body. When I say spiritual I mean your attitude toward yourself, other people, *and* your higher power.

Your permanent solution depends not on what you have to do to change but *who you will have to become in order to change*. You will begin to move forward; you may stall sometimes, and then you will move forward, often even faster than you were. But people move forward at varying rates. My most important breakthrough, waking up to a new positive me, took less than three months from the time I made it my goal. Regardless of how long it takes you, here is my promise: you can progress from merely surviving diabetes – that is, not dying early – to thriving. Life isn't merely to be endured, it's to be celebrated – shouted about until breathless. Who said that kind of glorious life is only for others?

Your mind may be telling you that you're managing diabetes just fine. You may be happy. If so, congratulations; you're in the minority. But are you happy, really? Here is one of the best kept secrets ever, although you might not like hearing it. Learning to embrace adversity is the secret to true happiness. When we accept our woundedness, rather than denying it, we begin to see things differently than when our concern is only with overcoming the wound. And once you've implemented your authentic code it won't feel a bit like adversity. You will no longer *suffer from diabetes*. Having diabetes will feel like no effort or trouble. And you'll have consistently low HA1c levels!*

The difference in your quality of life will amaze you. Have you ever thought you could actually thrive, even with diabetes? Maybe you have felt it once in a while. Or maybe not at all, but don't fret. If you have felt it, you have glimpsed what life can be for you. Have you ever felt you were put on Earth to learn an important lesson, and that once

*HA1c refers to the test that measures the level of hemoglobin A1c in the blood as a means of determining the average blood sugar concentrations for the preceding two or three months – called also A1c, HbA1c, glycated hemoglobin, glycohemoglobin, and glycosylated hemoglobin.

that lesson was learned you will finally fill a void within you? I did. And from that I've learned that most people feel the same void that has not been filled in spite of their efforts.

Having diabetes made me wake up. I was on a path of self-destruction – the slow death of my soul from spiritual malnourishment and beliefs that did not support me. In my stubborn state I wouldn't listen to people who wanted to help me. I always had to be right – my fragile self-esteem needed to believe I was right. Throughout these pages, the story of an utter turn around, my complete transformation, will unfold, and, hopefully, will free you. I hope to change in you whatever it is that is keeping you from living free and dancing through life with joy, not in spite of having diabetes, but while embracing it and yet grateful for who you are. This truth is what will fill the void.

This next part is a bit difficult to understand but try as best you can to imagine how my process works. You must become aware there is something missing – that something's wrong in your life. That's the DIS-ease. You may feel unhappy, exhausted, frustrated, apathetic, negative, or anything that comes to mind as your DIS-ease. If you don't understand this at first don't worry. All I am saying is that besides diabetes there is something deeper causing DIS-ease. There has to be. Otherwise you would be happily living your life, not frustrated and searching for answers.

Identifying this problem will help you to understand why you have DIS-ease. To decode it you will need to drill down beneath the beliefs, thoughts, feelings, and activities that contribute to it, and create a new environment in which what you think and feel fully supports who you are, what you do, and why you do it. Decoding your DIS-ease in this way will support being a happy and healthy person who has the *symptom* of diabetes, and it will take the sting out of having diabetes.

My wish is that people everywhere, with or without diabetes, will wake up to the real *why* behind our malady. People who are unaware that their lives can be much richer won't pick up this manual. If they do they may tell themselves it doesn't work. But when people have the courage to pick it up and begin the work, the awakening will energize them to the point where they see that the process is do-able. I hope that's you. I hope you are among those reading this who believes change is possible.

Part 1. The Beginning of Simplicity

It ain't what you don't know that gets you into trouble.
It's what you know for sure that just ain't so.

~Mark Twain

Chapter 1. Why this Book?

I have good problem-solving skills but I was stuck for a long time because I resented having to manage diabetes and hated every time I needed to test my blood sugar, take a shot of insulin, and avoid sugar. Forgive my immaturity at that stage of my life, but every time I thought about trying to find real solutions what always came up was, "But why me? Why should I have to deal with it? It isn't fair!" And it stopped me from solving my problem.

People with good organizational skills never seem to have that problem. If you have a good system for managing your diabetes, you test regularly, your HA1c results are in the sixes, and sometimes in the fives, and you're not sure if you need to read on, consider this: are you managing your illness because of the fear and anxiety you feel? Are will power and obedience keeping you on the straight and narrow? Regardless of your good control, you may not realize your energy is low. If this is you, most likely your doctor is pleased with your control. But that may be part of the problem; you may not realize you're irritated that you even *have* diabetes. Or if you do realize it you may not know that you can be free from frustration *and* have diabetes at the same time.

Whether or not you are in good control there is usually something mental or emotional that keeps your energy low and stops you from enjoying life. Are you doing what you've always dreamed of doing? Or did you stop, like I did, when you were diagnosed? You may have drawn a conclusion that your life will now consist of managing a disease. You may even be obsessed with control at the exclusion of everything else. You may not know it's possible to have diabetes *and* live a full and happy life. Today's technology eliminates the need to give up on your dreams. So if your system requires you to stop living in order to be in good control *it needs tweaking*. This book will help you find out whether or not your current code is working and will help you fix what isn't.

In the early years having diabetes was constantly on my mind. My thoughts went something like, "I shouldn't have eaten that… I shouldn't eat this (while I ate it)… I shouldn't think about eating that (then I ate it)… I should test my blood sugar… I didn't test it when I thought of it… (an hour later) I still haven't tested… I'm too tired… I'll test in the morning." Accompanying these thoughts was always that awful "G" word – guilt. And beneath that I was mad, resentful, isolated and lonely. I felt misunderstood and somehow inferior because I had diabetes – and moody, exasperated, and outraged.

At church one Sunday when I was new to the disease, something huge dawned on me. We attended a fundamentalist Christian Church. The pastor's message was based on a Biblical citation; we *are all dregs of the earth and there is not one good thing about us*; he was making the point that having Jesus in our hearts is that much more wonderful by comparison. Everyone said "Amen."

Like *pond scum*, I thought.

"There is nothing good about us," he said, and he emphasized *nothing*. He went on to open up to his congregation – to tell his story of abuse as a child, and how fortunate he had been to be saved by the Lord! He was indeed fortunate – and felt worthless. A part of me thought he was right – I felt like pond scum! But there was a deeper part of me that didn't agree. I knew I had been hiding and it was time to stop. And it was the beginning of the journey of a lifetime.

I hope you don't obstinately let your pain drag on like I did. My journey has been extended by my own unwillingness to move beyond anger to solutions. It took me another twenty years. My hope in documenting the lessons from the school of *suffering-from-diabetes*, is that you will have an easier time because of what I know. The way to do it is to stop right now trying to swim against the current.

Here is what I mean. We sabotage ourselves with our beliefs about how life is and how to approach it. What worked a few years ago doesn't work anymore. Here is how it should work and how self-sabotage disrupts the flow of growth. An event takes place. You respond. A change occurs. And you form a new behavior. So… an event occurs and you think a certain way about the event; you're either OK or you're not. If you're OK, great. You move on and it has not gotten in your way.

But if you aren't OK with the outcome you can become stuck. What made you stuck? Was it the event? No, it was your choices about the event – how you thought, felt, and acted in response to it. This is the vicious circle we all find ourselves in from time to time. When you have learned what you need to learn, and only then, you will be able to once again move forward in life. The lesson becomes engrained.

Doctors and dietitians tell you what to do. It isn't their job to tell you how – how to stay in control when you don't feel like it. For example, when you've had a bad day, your energy is gone and you feel like laying on the couch. Maybe you want a cupcake. For me there were deep issues beneath the surface of what was going on in my life that made me want that cupcake.

I'm not yet near the end of my journey, but within these pages I reveal the story of my gradual U-turn from destroying myself to living a life I could only dream about. It took diabetes to do it. I don't know what it otherwise would have taken for me to come into the full realization of who I am. Years ago I would have said my life was over. It's ironic that my life is full now because I have diabetes. It's the kind of transformation that makes a person grateful for whatever it was; whatever had to be taken away in order to learn something huge.

My Story

Some people think my openness about my own story might undermine my credibility while working as a mentor for others. It's true my style is unique compared to many mentors, but I think nothing could be further from the truth. My style has done more to help others overcome their own troubles than anything else I could do.

One client told me that what he liked best about me was my willingness to be human. He felt that my insight helped me understand him. When I am willing to *undress in front of others* so to speak, people more easily and willingly let down their own guard. They identify with me and they progress much further and faster. I am also well aware that millions of people have experienced traumatic events that they need to face; we are all essentially in parallel dramas.

The DIS-ease is mental

Psychologists say that at the moment of trauma a person, child or adult, abruptly stops maturing emotionally. If this statement is accurate it means I became emotionally stunted in pre-adolescence. That is, in order to bury the pain of child abuse I had to cut off the part of me that I did not want to acknowledge and bury it deep. They call it Post Traumatic Stress Disorder or PTSD. It's caused by the stress of trying to keep a lid on the pressure-cooker of emotions brought on by traumatic events—in my case abuse. The result stays with a child well into adulthood. It manifests in symptoms of depression and anxiety. It's what brought on diabetes for me.

Once I became an adult I slowly began unburying my DIS-ease. But it wasn't easy. In fact, I didn't know that that was what I needed to do. I had symptoms of anxiety and depression but most of the time I wasn't even aware of them. I was very good at hiding my problems even from myself. But before I could begin I would first have to learn how to acknowledge the symptoms.

According to the American Institute of Stress, to name one authority on stress, many emotional and physical disorders have been linked to stress. They include depression, anxiety, heart attacks, stroke, hypertension, immune system disturbances that increase susceptibility to infections, a host of virally-linked disorders ranging from the common cold and herpes to AIDS and certain cancers, as well as autoimmune diseases like rheumatoid arthritis and multiple sclerosis. In addition stress can have direct effects on the skin (rashes, hives, and dermatitis), the gastrointestinal system (GERD, peptic ulcer, irritable bowel syndrome, and ulcerative colitis), the endocrine system (diabetes), and can contribute to insomnia and degenerative neurological disorders like Parkinson's disease. In fact, it's hard to think of any disease in which stress does not play an aggravating role or any part of the body that is not affected. The table on the following page reflects some of the symptoms chronic stress victims suffer. The list continues to grow as the extensive ramifications of stress are increasingly being appreciated.

Looking over this list I realize I had nearly seventy-five symptoms of anxiety and depression and I didn't think there was very much wrong with me! For a while I believed everybody had the complaints I had. I *decided* to believe that everyone suffers from these symptoms, but some people are just better than me at pretending they don't have them. *I'll just have to do a better job,* I thought. So at first, rather than address my problems, I buried them deeper and became an expert at hiding. That decision cost me in many ways – in the time I could have spent really living *and* in the cost to my health.

Why would anyone choose dying over living? Because they're not aware it's what they're choosing. They believe they are choosing life. After all, what is the alternative? Bringing up all the stinky filth buried long ago? I'll tell you why you should bring up all the stinking filth.

The first thing I learned on my path to wellness was that I was suffering, not living. I was suffering needlessly. Next I realized I had been wearing nagging self-loathing like a familiar old coat; smelly, tattered, yet so comfortable I wasn't even aware I was wearing it. And I learned that this *me* that was all I knew was a false *me*. What I didn't know was that while there were plenty of people suffering alongside me with their own buried piles of crap, there were plenty more who weren't.

Allergies	Worthlessness	Fear of what others think
Body tremors	Loneliness	Excessively defensive
Exhausted	Decreased sex drive	Self-consciousness
Clumsy	Frequent headaches	Trouble Communicating
Lightheaded	High startle reflex	Rapid speech
Irritable	Shortness of breath	Difficulty concentrating
Unable to relax	Forgetfulness	Stuck thoughts
Overwhelmed	Fear of losing control	Emotionally flat/numb
Racing heart	Impending doom	Flu-like symptoms
Fidgety	Overloaded	TMJ from clenching
Impulse buying	Insomnia	Angry and hostile
Night sweats	Ringing in the ears	Social withdrawal
Déjà Vu	Desensitization	Dramatic mood swings
Panic attacks	Fear of dying	Lack of patience
Disorientation	Nightmares	Increased appetite
Teeth grinding	Incessant mind chatter	Decreased appetite
Chronic worry	Social anxiety	Emotional detachment
Powerlessness	Stuttering/stammering	Severe frustration
Suicidal	Feeling spaced out	Difficulty deciding

Nervousness	Feelings of unreality	Neck/shoulder stiffness
Guilt	Depersonalization	Disturbing dreams
Chronic pressure	Overreaction	Difficulty learning
Racing thoughts	Frequent crying	Lying/making excuses
Shame	Underlying fear	Crying for no reason

(Common symptoms of stress)

The good news is happiness is real and everyone can have it. Once I understood I didn't have to suffer I could begin to get better. It was like I had always known it but had only recently awakened to it – like Dorothy and her ruby slippers, the way back was there all along.

Why wouldn't you want to be free from a terrible burden once you have recognized it – and once you see you can put it down? Because it's simple but not as easy as it looks. Here are three important facts.

- That false *me* was the only identity I knew
- Letting go of the only identity a person has known is the hardest thing to do; you feel as if you are going *down the rabbit hole*
- The best way to start to heal is to find a way to begin

It's amazing that once you find out what you need, your path will lead you to getting it. Mine led me to a mentor who knew I needed to learn what unconditional love *feels* like. I'm talking about mattering in a real way by a person whose reason to be in your life is to help you heal.

My mentor, a Methodist minister named David Butler, said, "You need to know you matter to just one other person." His statement was about modeling unconditional love, the kind of pure love I had never known before. It was the beginning of healing for me. Once I felt

I truly mattered to someone I knew cared about me I began to matter to myself. Just like David said I would.

What's Stopping You?

It took me more than thirty years to finally realize I was getting in my own way. We all do it – self sabotage. For me it was a gnawing feeling in my chest and stomach that I didn't really matter that made me realize it. So I became a people pleaser. What others wanted was always more important to me than what I wanted. It helped fill the gap whenever I had someone to do something for. For a while at least.

And I realized that as adults my siblings and I couldn't have been more distant. When we were children it was too frightening to talk about it. There was a lot we did not want to know. We further distanced ourselves as adults, each going in separate directions. Our mother had died several years before and we only saw each other at our father's house, where things were always tense.

Going to my dad's house made me anxious; he might do or say something that would embarrass us all, or worse, would compromise my kids. Outwardly our father was a knowledgeable parent who had raised six children to successful adulthood. But in truth we were lost, he was lost, and the path we were on only enabled us all to stay stuck in our own messes.

As a child I was not taught my value. In the absence of this important teaching children will reason they are *not* valuable. Ego is a fragile thing in children, and parents, aunts, cousins and schoolmates, and strangers can easily take away a child's value and not even realize they're doing it. I believe that people who don't like themselves have been unknowingly taught they are not important. Then as adults it becomes almost impossible to believe in the concept of self-love, especially without outside help. And if they don't have self-love how can they possibly teach it to their kids? It's no wonder self-esteem is so low when kids graduate from high school. And this feeling of unworthiness bleeds over into all areas of life.

The first defect I began to be aware of was my people pleaser tendency and the fact that I didn't care about myself and I didn't think I really mattered to anyone else.

What sabotages you and stops you from moving toward happiness? You may be stuck in fear that your life holds no meaning. Or fear diabetes and other illnesses will bring on worse illnesses. Afraid your life is over. You may be just plain mad like I was – mad at self, parents, and God. Or you may still grieve the loss of your vitality. Like losing a parent or a child you still may be in mourning for your lost health. All these emotions rob you of your energy and there is only one thing to do; face them and tackle them one at a time. In part Two we will look at the role emotions play in vitality. First let's look at the obvious physical aspects, as well as some less obvious ones.

The Effects of Stress on Health

You may not agree that all diabetes occurs due to stress but here is one universal truth: most disease is reflective of some physical or mental condition that has gone untreated long enough to manifest in symptoms. It's often a reflection of how you feel, think, and act – how you feel about yourself, how you treat yourself, how much you love, like, or dislike yourself, how you view the world, and how you treat others. It's a message to pay attention. It could be that you have always had low self-esteem and just didn't know it. Nobody wants to acknowledge they don't like themselves. That is why low self-esteem is such a scourge and why it wreaks havoc with our lives and with our health. In a moment we will take you through a series of simple questions designed to help you find out how much you love or don't love yourself.

Whether you believe it or not, if you hate having diabetes it is an unhealthy mental condition. If you believe diabetes is a death sentence then that's what it will be for you – a self-fulfilling prophecy. If you look at diabetes as a ball and chain, chaining you to a miserable future, then it will be just that. And if it is a death sentence to you, like it was for me, you will not be at all happy about managing it. Your doctor will teach you proper self-care, but you may tell yourself almost anything to keep from having to face and deal with the monster. Or you will follow your doctor's advice to the letter and feel tied to it like a ball and chain, hoping science will eventually free you by handing you a cure.

We wear our stories like a badge, declaring, "Look at what I am surviving," and all the while we feel instead like we're dying. What you need is a new story you can feel better about – happier about.

The strong correlation of Type 2 diabetes and obesity alone shows us that something is very wrong. While there are genetic factors at play I propose that what's wrong usually begins with your thinking. Just look at the connection between obesity and low self-esteem.

Modern research shows that your cells know and reflect what is going on in your mind. Even when you aren't consciously aware there is anything wrong! Science is just beginning to make the connection between illness and psychology, although doctors have been perplexed by the placebo effect for more than fifty years. Personally, while I have not been able to jump-start my pancreas to produce insulin, I rarely catch colds and flu, a huge change from just a few years ago, and I attribute it to my improved life-approach.

Why you are ill is the key that will help you unlock your wellness. I consider all illness to contain a message from your body to your conscious mind that there is something wrong in your whole self and it's not going away until you consciously work through it.

Seems crazy to me

Here is a perfect example of how all this works. As I was preparing to embark on a new path in my life I realized how daunting it was. I have been an employee of other organizations for so long I don't know how to build income for myself. I am not entrepreneurial. For me it was incredibly scary and although I have mentored hundreds of others to take the leap, to *free-fall*, I was not actually a willing participant in this *free-fall* method.

The potential pitfalls made me numb, the first of which being *no money*. I thought it made sense to find a job while I was developing my practice, but no one was hiring. Maybe I was too old or too over-qualified, but I kept plugging away at it.

One morning I broke my leg while getting ready to go for a job interview. My first thought as I sat on the bathroom floor looking at my left leg, which was sticking out sideways at the knee, was *Why are you going in a direction opposite of the direction you are meant go?* And I instantly knew it was not really me thinking this – it was a spiritual thought. My leg was sticking out to the side, a position that reflected the strategy I was using to get to my goal – going sideways. I often listen to my higher power, but I do admit that at that time in my life I found I was obstinate about listening... that is until I got hit over the head with a broken leg! Life, or God, has a way of bringing us back around to what's necessary.

Physical, emotional, mental, and spiritual stress

Let's look at some of the types of stress we experience. *Physical stressors* that can help bring on diabetes include stressful personal relationships, stressful jobs, poverty, illness, lack of direction, and health concerns such as obesity and depression. Stressors need to be dealt with and resolved or they will create physical symptoms. And if some stress contributed to diabetes in the first place you can bet it will continue to cause you problems. Physical stressors may be brought on by mental ones, such as self-doubt, thinking you're not smart enough, or thinking you deserve the bad thing that's happening. These stressors are reinforced by emotional stressors – the feelings accompanying the thoughts that are stressing you out.

The stressors that contributed to my onset fall into four categories; physical, mental, emotional, and spiritual stress. At onset I was just about to turn thirty, yet my diabetes is the childhood type. They call it LADA, or *Latent Autoimmune Diabetes in Adults*. I am certain it was brought on by stress, and if I could have a do-over, I would deal with my stress more proactively. I believe I could have avoided diabetes altogether.

One burden that contributed, I think, was a chronic sinus infection I'd had since age twelve. I had broken my nose and it had gone untreated, which resulted in complete nasal blockage. To complicate that I had hay fever that was among the highest my doctors have ever seen, and one long sinus infection that lasted twenty years. Researchers believe that Type 1 diabetes is often caused by an over active immune system which attacks the pancreas and kills the insulin producing islet cells. One sign of an overly efficient immune system is severe allergies. As well, a chronic infection lowers the body's ability to fight disease. And that was just one source of my stress.

My major mental stress was my job. I had worked for a government agency where people stood in line for up to two hours watching us work and waiting for their turn. By the time a person got to my counter he was at a boiling point, which was when he would take his frustration out on me. Years of that were taking their toll and I knew it because I carried it home with me; and took out my frustration on my poor husband.

My spiritual stress was simply that I didn't know what I was good at, if anything. I felt my mediocre job reflected my mediocre life. I was unsatisfied. I know now that this had a lot to do with low self-esteem. The most effective thing I have done in my battle with disease was to own that I did not really love, or even like, myself. Spiritual stress occurs when people don't properly nurture their souls; their lives hold very little meaning.

The biggest stress I lived with was that I was shut down emotionally with chronic depression that I was hiding from myself and the world. Some depression is brought on by trauma and the experiences that induce PTSD. I learned I had been emotionally stunted around age ten and constantly suppressing it had led to chronic depression that followed me well into adulthood and stayed until I addressed it.

Low Self-Value

Call it low confidence, low self-worth, or doubts about your usefulness as a human being. If you want to finally know whether or not you have low self-worth I can help you. Children and adults in our culture, as in many cultures, are not typically taught that healthy self-esteem is essential for survival. Our culture, for one, tends to teach kids to not value themselves. But in fact, the academic world, families and marriages, corporations, all work environments, healthy governments, and the health of the world economy all depend on healthy individual self-esteem for success. Your happiness depends on it too. Your parents may have hugged you and spoken soft words, and that may have felt like it was enough. More often, though, it wasn't enough.

A good friend once told me we need four hugs a day just for maintenance, but at least twelve for good health. I don't know how statistical those numbers are, but the more hugs I get in a day the better my day goes. How many hugs do you give and receive? It has been said that one in four people do not have a single person we trust enough to share our hurts and pain. How many true friends do you have?

A short self-esteem assessment

I invite you to privately take a short self-esteem assessment. Using a blank sheet of paper, answer these questions. Be honest and loving to yourself as you sort through it.

1. How often do you think about yourself throughout the average day? Write down the first number that comes to mind.

2. When you think of yourself, what is the nature of the thought? Is it usually something you did that was good and that you are proud of? Something you did that will help you grow? On the flip side, it could be something like: That was bad, that was stupid, that was selfish, I am selfish, or even, I am useless. Use your best analytical skills to come up with exact statements you regularly tell yourself (it can be even more telling to keep a notebook by you and write them down as they come to you over a 24-hour period).

3. What does the term *unconditional* love mean to you? If you always love your children no matter what they do, that's unconditional. If you love them only when they're good, it's conditional love. Now take a look at yourself. Do you always love yourself no matter what? Conditional or unconditional? It's a simple, but not a very easy, question. Your complete honesty will make it clear.

4. Do you love yourself as much as you love the people you care about? Compare the difference between how much you love your children, your wife or husband, and your parents with how much you love yourself. Be completely honest.

5. Now look at your religious teachings. Would any truly spiritual ideal teach that you are less worthy of love than anyone else? According to your beliefs, is it right to love yourself? Or is it selfish? If it were up to you what would you choose to believe about self-love, regardless of what your religion seems to teach?

People are often surprised to find there is a double standard to their love. Of course they say they always love their kids, no matter what. But they don't say the same about themselves. When I ask that question people usually fall silent.

This, then, is where to begin. Close your eyes and ask yourself, on a scale of one to ten, one being *I loathe my very existence*, and ten being *I feel as though I can stand up to anything and I can do anything I put my mind to.*

- A number between one and four indicates a degree of *low self-esteem.*
- Five through seven says you believe you are no better and no worse than other people.
- If you honestly said eight, nine, or ten your life has meaning.

Start with the number you chose. If you aren't happy with your number, ask the questions every day and do the work necessary to raise it. Your answers may vary each time you ask the questions because self-esteem is intensely tied to how you feel in the moment you ask. When I start believing I don't know what I am doing with regard to how to make a living creating a business my number goes down. The people in your life can cause the number to go up or down too, depending on how much you believe what they say to and about you.

What you can do

My severe allergic reactions caused by an unhealthy hyper-active immune system and a genetic predisposition to diabetes made me susceptible. But looking back, when I piled on high job-related stress and chronic depression for over twenty years it seems it was inevitable. To truly heal you need to uncover the sources of the unhealthiness in your life.

Regardless of what life has thrown at you, and regardless of the direction in which your life takes you, you must gather the courage to face and deal with it. You can either let it stop you from moving forward *or* you can see it as your next step.

I had a friend who lost a child to SIDs. She was always *fine* about having only one child, but, she would say, "Everyone else has a problem with it. Everyone tells me I really should try to have another child." When someone keeps talking about the same issue for fifteen years I know they are carrying it with them but not working through it to get to the other side of what has become their wall. The story she told herself was that when her second baby died she dealt with it and moved on. She told herself it was everyone else who had a problem. What she needed was a better story – a story that works. Something like, *I am sad you are gone from me but I'm happy that I knew you.* Figure it out rather than burying it. Your story is part of who you are and it always will be. However, it does not define you in any way.

You have probably guessed by now that low energy is the result of heavy emotions that are likely so much a part of your life you hardly notice them. Positive emotions – courage, acceptance, and love – do not contribute to poor diabetes control. There is no way they possibly could. Instead your objective ought to be to feel and then move on (not repressing) from any and all negative emotions you feel, and replace them as best you can with positive ones. That's easier said than done, but we will show you an easy way to change the way you feel. Not all at once, but you will be surprised at how you feel in just a week, then in six months.

There is purpose to each of our lives. Some people know it from childhood but others live their entire lives and never find it. My real purpose in life didn't become clear to me until I was in my fifties. It started with learning to love myself, and once I did that I began the process of deciding not to hate the journey I was on. During that time I took some important steps toward changing a multitude of beliefs that were keeping me unhappy. Then, once I changed a dozen or so of my limiting beliefs an incredible thing happened!

My authentic blueprint took shape – a system perfect for managing my disease with no trouble at all; one that allows me to be healthy *and* happy at the same time. Now diabetes is something I take care of in my day because it's time to; just like I fix dinner, do the dishes, and read my emails. It has no sting now. I don't have to love it; I just want to feel neutral and not hate it. I no longer feel anything negative when I think about it, and that helps me take a lot better care of myself.

My new realizations and my new code are the soul of my message. It became clear that I need to practice my code every day and teach my methods. My new code consists of a plan I follow every day in each of four important areas of my life. I will show you my particular code later. For now I want to lay the groundwork.

The Four Facets of Living with Diabetes

Practical. The practical aspect of diabetes includes the obvious; actions you take based on information your doctor and other health care providers give you, as well as information you research to help you control the physical symptoms of your disease. This includes your tools, diet components, carbohydrate counting, blood sugar testing, exercise, an insulin pump if applicable, and living a healthy lifestyle. Practical aspects also include things you do for your soul. It's been said by many philosophers that the body is the physical manifestation of the soul. Soulful activities lower your blood pressure and heart rate. These activities include anything you love to do, that, while you are doing it you tend to lose yourself in it, to the point that you can easily lose track of time. These activities help keep you positive and happy. Including them will bring you balance, much needed for being at peace in your body, which will give you better control, too.

Mental. Mental attributes of diabetes care include how and what you think and know about diabetes; additional knowledge about diabetes management, health, and diet; periodicals, and books; and learning more and better ways to manage diabetes. And it includes your memories and the things you tell yourself.

Emotional. The emotional facet includes how you feel about diabetes; how anger, resentment, guilt, fear, and apathy affect you when it comes to living with diabetes. How joy and love can help you gain better control. And how you feel about yourself, diabetes, your roles, and your life.

Spiritual. Spiritually, think about all your beliefs; about God, religion, other people, yourself, your body, and your life.

Through a series of fortunate events I was able to learn the dynamics of life coaching and I found I was very good at helping people see what they need to do to get where they want to go. But the most important result of my training was what it did for me. I have always felt I could impact others' lives. What I did not know was how much learning to help others heal would heal me. I found the four important facets of an amazing system, and using that I developed the perfect structure for me – what I call my authentic diabetes code.

When we teach we learn and when I pointed out to a client what she needed to do next there were always three fingers pointing back at me. I needed to be willing to do what I was asking her to do. And I believe I have a responsibility to help others with the same help I have been given. What we learn becomes a road map that others can use. I hope that showing you my map will make things easier for you. And if it's easier you will have a greater likelihood of succeeding.

The method I am giving you here is quite a short cut from the twenty or so years it took me; you can avoid my mistakes by simply knowing what mistakes I made and not making them. A map gives people direction and clarity so they spend less time in confusion. And the most important aspect of having a good map is that it can be incredibly motivating. There's light at the end of the dark tunnel. You're not the only person with this problem. There is a solution. And you can do it! Remember though; while it is a short-cut it will still take some time and energy, mostly in the beginning.

First, you need to hear "You can do it" more than anything else. People spend a lot of energy talking ourselves out of things for more reasons than I can name. You need to read "You can do it" from me, hear "You can do it" from people who care about you, and say "I can do it" to yourself. And you need all this regularly. My mentor David cared enough about me to help me through my dark tunnel. It was an entirely new concept to have someone so intensely concerned about my well-being, and the first time I allowed someone to have that role in my life. He told me "You can do it" all the time. I needed that, especially at first, because my own doubt questioned every thought, every feeling, and every action.

Even though chances are we have never met I care about you in the same way. My guiding principle is *Where ever I go, whomever I meet, I make sure people know they matter*. It's core to us as human beings. And here is what else I know:

- Unhappiness erodes lives
- The human mind is a tough battleground
- You can turn unhappiness into happiness
- It's available for every living being
- *You can do it*

I love seeing real, positive, lasting change in people. My greatest joy is celebrating with someone who is overcoming low self-esteem, anger, pain, perfectionism, and the rest of the garbage in his or her life. They've come alive. They can hardly speak they are so overcome with joy.

Who in your life cares about you? If you don't have anyone find someone. At the very least I hope my telling you helps you care more about yourself. At that point the other people will show up for you.

Chapter 2. What Decoding Diabetes Means

Learning is not child's play; we cannot learn without pain.
~ Aristotle

Success is in the Details

I cannot guess what it will take for you; I know only the steps I needed to take for me to become happy and healthy with diabetes. Many of your steps will be different, but you will want to use my tools and processes as they will help. Within these pages are principles to help you take your steps. Guiding principles are timeless laws that help you make decisions that will bring the best possible outcomes. There are thousands of principles in nature, all helpful for solving different kinds of problems. Throughout this book I will present principles that I have found to be the most helpful for the physical, mental, emotional, social, and spiritual aspects of being human, for myself as well as the hundreds of people I have helped. They are all relevant to living happily with diabetes.

Your beliefs affect your success

You are what you continually think. I am sure you know it's true, but do you know how paralyzing and limiting your beliefs can be when they are not in your best interest? When animals make a mistake they learn to live with the result (if they don't die from the mistake). Humans are the only organisms that punish themselves for making mistakes. Humans show an amazing capacity to punish ourselves for years for just one decision that had an outcome we interpreted as negative.

Our species alone has the capacity to remember mistakes and mentally relive them, beating ourselves up and obsessing about them over and over again. Our memory is so good we will do this to ourselves for weeks, months, and even years. Your spouse, parents, children, siblings, neighbors, friends, and even your boss help you remember too. Often they won't let you ever forget it. The reminders you hear from within and outside of you reinforce beliefs that already existed – beliefs that limit your happiness; often beliefs that created your unhappiness in the first place.

Most people just want to complain. Only three percent are ever going to do anything to change their ineffective behaviors. Ninety seven percent want to stay where it's comfortable. But why would people keep their lives as they are, even when they are unhappy? Deep down most people don't really believe they can change these behaviors very much. Most people find it's easier to come up with a reason not to move than to move – because it's easier. What will it take to change the results you are getting? What will it take to make the difficult choice? If you are in the three percent, congratulate yourself!

Give yourself permission to let this be a process

You have thousands of beliefs unconsciously governing you. Some are working for you and some are not. Many of the beliefs have been in control for a long time; some of them for years or decades. You're not going to change them quickly. Permanent change cannot occur easily and quickly – not in the face of decades of old beliefs. Some of the beliefs are false. I want you to understand that their power over you is only that you think they're true.

But many of them are not; they're stories you agreed to long ago. Beliefs like, "I can't do it," "It's too hard," "It won't help," and "This won't work." A few of my personal stories were "I'm not important," "I'm worthless," "I can't control my blood sugar," "My energy will always be low," and "I hate diabetes." Do you have any of these? I have permanently changed all of the beliefs I held onto for decades that weren't serving me. And I still work to change old beliefs when I find they aren't helping.

When you come across something in this book or in life that "sticks" with you, understand that it is a core component of your ideal system – something you need to adopt and adapt to your life. You may have difficulty believing you can incorporate it easily and effortlessly, but you can. You can even change the belief that you can't do it to you *can* do it. I'll show you how easy it is.

For years I believed taking care of diabetes is hard and takes too much time away from enjoying life. I had classic either/or conditioning and it made diabetes a constant irritation. As long as I felt that way about it I stayed frustrated and hurt. I would frequently put off testing or eating right in favor of what I wanted to be doing instead. When I did think of doing something I didn't want to do that was good for me the old anger would rear up and keep me from acting responsibly. That paradigm kept my blood sugars consistently high.

The hardest part of changing a belief is becoming aware that you *want* to change it. For me the most difficult belief to change was that I am worth the effort. But I learned how to change that belief and once I did I found other beliefs I wanted to change too. I wanted beliefs that served me instead. "I effortlessly and easily control my blood sugars." "My blood sugars are always in the target range when I get up in the morning." "I always know the correct dosage of insulin to take." "I don't have lows in the middle of the night." "Taking care of diabetes is easy."

And my life changed. I found myself remembering to test, testing, and then going on with my life like it was nothing. I found it is no more trouble than making the bed, squeegeeing the shower, or fixing a sandwich – no more trouble than maintaining my life. And when I thought about testing, the old nagging resentment just wasn't there anymore! I effectively *took the wind out of the sails* of hating diabetes. I intuitively hear a number in my head and that's my dose. When I get up in the morning it's in the target range. I brought my HA1c results from eight or higher to consistently in the sixes. And it doesn't take one thing away from my life style. In fact, I'm able to do more because my energy is a lot higher.

Begin to compile a list of beliefs that are the most important for you to change. Keep track of it, keep it handy, and add to it as you think of more. Use the note pages at the back of this book, inside the front cover, or on the front page of your journal. If you want, put them into categories, physical, mental, emotional, and spiritual. If you don't know which category they belong to don't worry about it.

Here are a few examples of some system components that showed up for me as my code developed, and their categories.

- This disease is too hard on my family.
  Category: Spiritual

- I crave sweets, candy, and especially bread.
  Category: Physical and emotional

- I can't remember when or how much my last dose was.
  Category: Mental

- I can't decide whether or not to go on a pump.
  Category: Physical and mental

- There is no way to not hate diabetes
  Category: Emotional

- How can God love me if He allowed this?
  Category: Spiritual

Remember to give yourself time for the ideas to develop. It may seem like a lot of work but it will get easier.

You have all the components of your ideal blueprint inside you. Don't worry if the solutions don't come to you right away. I have many techniques to help you identify and develop them. You never know when your solutions will show up so be ready to capture and keep track of them.

How You Deal with Things is How You Deal with Disease

Understanding your personality is like having the exact recipe for the life you want. It tells you what to expect from yourself when you're not feeling good or you've had some unpleasant turn of events. Have you ever noticed that you are at your worst when you're not feeling good? I have a lazy streak and when my blood sugar is off, when I am tired, I get lazier. When you think, feel, and do things you're not proud of, your energy is at its lowest and you are at your worst.

Your personality also tells you where you shine, and what you do that's helping you and those you love. Before I learned I have talent and passion I had never tapped into I did mediocre work in every job I had. However, I did exemplary work on my own projects. Because I loved doing them I was good at them.

If it's not tied to what I love I will do a mediocre, or even a poor job, or I'll quit early into a project and move on to the next thing – the next "bright, shiny object." Are you beginning to see my personality

27

type? Unless I love the process, I lose interest and the next project always has more appeal than what I'm working on; in other words, my current project will die.

Cooking is like that for me, and watching my favorite movies while knitting. It was when I discovered I have a talent for mentoring and teaching people who are looking for answers that I found new motivation; I have never wanted to move on from coaching. That's because I finally found what I was looking for. I was able to finally find my true passion because I was able to take enough risk to find it. I wanted it enough to trust myself enough to go after it – enough to not worry about failing.

My point is I found facets of my personality I don't particularly like and others that have made me good at certain things. Knowing what motivates you is crucial to understanding what you need that's different from the next person's needs.

One book on personality, *The People Code*, by Taylor Hartman (Hartman, 1997), has served me over the years better than any other. It helps me understand the difference between my personality and how I am affected by my past and present environments. You came into the world hard-wired. Whether you came in kicking and screaming or calm and peaceful depended on your personality. Your environment and your genetics combined to shape who you are and they continue to shape you. This is why two people perceive the world so differently, which is important to understand when it comes to diabetes. It explains why some people deal with diabetes with ease, while it's jarring for others, and to some it never gets any easier.

There is an energetic side and a tired side to your personality. When you're tired, characteristics come out that you don't like. This unhealthiness is often physical, especially if you have a chronic illness like diabetes, but emotional, mental, and spiritual unwell-ness affects you the same as physical illness. You may notice that when you feel better "bad" behaviors disappear without even thinking about it.

I am not very motivated by outcomes; I am motivated by processes. Positive outcomes are great but they are not my key motivators. Your motivators are the personality traits you were born with that drive your thoughts, perceptions, beliefs, and actions. You can make changes to behaviors but not to what motivates you. You will see that the changes you need to make that conflict with your personality lie outside your comfort zone and require a lot more conscious effort.

Hartman identifies four categories that motivate us primarily: joy, power, love, and peace. People usually have a dominant motivator and a combination of one or two of the others. We will discuss them briefly. You will probably identify your core motivator in the descriptions below.

Joy. My primary motivator has always been; What's going to be the most fun? This type of person lives carefree and "in the moment." However, we are easily distracted by anything that promises to be more fun than other tasks on a *to-do* list, especially when our energy is low. The other day I finally cleaned my bathroom. It was because the alternative was to do my taxes! This is something about me that I know; something more enjoyable distracts me and I forget to go back to the thing I was doing. So you can see why I was getting such poor results when I knew I needed to stop and take care of diabetes. Almost anything was preferable!

People motivated by having fun have trouble achieving goals. Think of the movie *Arthur*. To quit drinking his goal had to be his top priority, and even then he wavered a lot before he could commit. For joy-driven people goals must be tied to the heart's desire; the stronger they feel about their desires the better they are going to be at achieving them. They would rather think of goals as dreams or desires because a *goal* feels like it's going to be a lot of *work* (a word not found in the joyful person's vocabulary); it feels like it's going to be *no fun*. If you are motivated by joy, figure out how to take the sting out of having diabetes like I did. You can decide not to hate something if you work through the details. It will keep your energy high, which helps with your maintenance. And having better control will do wonders for achieving other dreams.

Power. People who are motivated by power are always thinking about time; they're always out of time and they feel there is never enough time. A person like this tends to be a thinker more than a feeler, which simply means they are more comfortable in the left hemisphere of their brains. If you are power-driven you may have issues with work/life balance. When people are determined to excel they often don't give themselves enough free time. They have a need to always be doing something or they think they are lazy. *Lazy* is a very bad word to them. They don't tend to feel entitled to or deserving of free time; they often feel impatient just sitting down for a few minutes.

Power people don't have time to be sick and they become extremely impatient when illness keeps them from pursuing and achieving their goals. Surprisingly, they have an easier time than other personality types controlling diabetes, but it's irritating for them because it gets in their way. To find balance, power people must add characteristics that are not part of their personality. For instance, they are able to relax and rejuvenate guilt-free as long as they don't think of it as being *lazy*.

Love. Would you believe that people motivated by love are the unhappiest people of all? They have the most depression, commit the most suicide, and have the lowest self-esteem of all personality types. They may have a higher incidence of diabetes as well. Loving others and being loved is the only thing that matters, but more than any other type of people they fail to understand the concept of self-love. They are plagued by perfectionism and future, and especially past, thinking. They hold on to memories, and that blocks their ability to move forward. True, awareness comes with these experiences, but they often wear their story like a badge of courage.

They are the true "feelers" of the world and are uncomfortable operating in the left hemisphere of their brains – the analytical side. They like creative, right-brained thinking. People motivated by love have a hard time letting go of their feelings and often find it impossible to be present. They feel powerless because to feel powerful they would have to feel in control of their emotions, and they almost never feel they have control of their emotions. If you're motivated by love, love yourself by honoring your own courage and yet staying objective about it as best you can. If you identify with this group you could say to yourself, *I have a story but I am not my story.* At that moment you will realize you can begin to move forward while still looking at the memory, grateful for what it has taught you. You will benefit by repeating to yourself often, s*tay present.*

Peace. People motivated by peace are good at letting things roll off their backs. They are great followers and they are usually more comfortable letting others make important decisions because they are uncomfortable making decisions. These people likely manage diabetes better because they have no difficulty following the doctor's instructions to the letter without question. In fact they thrive in such an environment. They are obedient by nature.

If this is you why are you reading this? If there is a personality engineered to manage diabetes and not hate it, it is the peacemakers. You are already an expert at details. You were born to develop and use systems and even to teach them to others. If you are motivated by peace and calmness and if you are still reading it's probably because one or more of the other motivators is motivating you. Remember, we have more than one core motivator.

Understanding what motivates you at your core is central to developing your authentic code. It will help you find what you're good at and what you need to work on when it comes to taking the sting out of having diabetes.

Solving Your Dilemma

Let's get started on the steps for solving your health dilemma. These are general steps we will use to specifically deal with diabetes. This system also works for other health issues you may be facing. If you're like me you like to have steps to follow when you're trying to do things differently. It's normal to hesitate when confronted with something new. But you may have already worked through a number of these steps. If so, congratulate yourself!

Your spirituality is a good place to begin; if you're not happy with your control you may be trying to do the physical without first solving a spiritual dilemma. We have talked about what I mean by spirituality; it's comprised of your beliefs about and your relationships with yourself, including your health, your higher power, and other people. If one or more of these is not right you are spiritually unbalanced, and that's costing you physical, mental, and emotional power over your disease.

Spiritual Steps

1. Take responsibility for your disease. Not necessarily for why you have it, but for what you will do about it. While you're at it, take responsibility for your emotions too, as best you can.
2. Be brutally honest. This is both the most difficult *and* the most important task. If you are new to the idea and you are frustrated it may be due to an unwillingness to be truthful with yourself.
3. Be patient. You will improve in your ability to be brutally honest with yourself.
4. Be your own coach. Everybody is a coach. It's our job to be our best coach; we are not in life to be our own worst critic.

Mental Steps

1. Gain knowledge you don't have. Be open to it. Subscribe to periodicals, read books, and join groups and online forums.

2. Pay attention to new developments that can make your life even better. My life completely changed when I found an iPhone app to track my glucose. It's less for me to have to keep track of so living with diabetes became very easy for me.

3. Pay attention to the things you tell yourself. Are they helping you or hurting you? Take notes. This information will be helpful for the emotional steps you can start to take.

Emotional Steps

1. Chronic joyless emotions come from the things people tell us and the things we tell ourselves. What you feel is the key to understanding what you're hearing inside your head. If you feel bad, sad, angry, bitter, guilty, or anything else that zaps your energy, do your best to capture the thought that caused the feeling.

2. Turn every undesirable thought around to create an opposite positive statement. If you don't believe it, write it down anyway.

3. Repeat the new thought every time the undesirable one shows up. We will show you how to do this in more detail.

Physical Steps

1. Make a list of your current physical problems and break it down into components.

2. Give serious thought to the advice and support you get from your doctor or nurse practitioner, your educators, and your dietitian. If you don't agree with them voice it. And search out other professionals to help you.

3. Take an active role in your diabetes treatment by asking better questions and contributing to your treatment.

4. Think critically about your care providers: do they support you? Do they hear you? Do you feel like you matter? Or does it seem like you're just a number in an endless line of sick people passing through their offices?

My Old and New Diabetes Codes

My problem	My broken old system
Low blood sugar in the evening	I didn't know why it was low *and* I did not want to be bothered
Fairly frequent middle-of-the-night lows, about every two months	I kept my BS high at night to avoid morning lows and then had high BS in the morning
High HA1c averages of 8 or 9	Didn't change; felt guilty about it
Blood Sugar tests frequently high	Guilt, futile attempts at self-discipline
Infrequent testing	Recrimination, more attempts at will-power
Low energy	Nothing I tried worked
High blood sugar upon waking	Couldn't solve without middle-of-the-night lows
Blood sugar fluctuations; spikes and severe lows	I tried the Insulin Pump but found I could not use it
Embarrassed about diabetes; feeling inferior	Conscious effort to be more relaxed about diabetes
Angry at God and asking why	Better acceptance but it still nagged at me

My problem	My broken old system
Lazy about taking care of it	I told myself I had good control and I was fine
I hated having diabetes	I put off testing because it reminded me how much I hated having diabetes
I did not truly love myself	I was gradually doing better
Diet high in simple carbohydrates	Reduced processed carbohydrates

This table and the one on the next page show the problems I had immediately before I made profound changes in my life. By that time my control was better than it had been in the past but my energy was still low and my system was still broken. These were physical issues and symptoms of my DIS-ease.

Be sure to identify things from each of the four areas so you know you have covered all your bases. You will not have your *authentic code* column yet because you are going to build it using this process. You will see from the table in the next page that I was gradually able to solve for each of my problems. I want to illustrate here what my system looks like as it continues to evolve. As you uncover your truth you will find other issues and you will want to add them.

My Problem	My Broken Old System	My Authentic Code	Note
Low blood sugar in the evening	I didn't know why it was low *and* I did not want to be bothered	I found I need larger boluses between waking and 2:00 PM and smaller ones from 2:00 to bedtime	More knowledge about how Lantus works and how my body responds to insulin
Fairly frequent middle-of-the-night lows, about every two months	I kept my BS high at night to avoid morning lows and then had high BS in the morning.	Better control and diet means my average BS level doesn't need to be high at bedtime.	I know the dose I need and I trust my intuition to *tell* me.
High HA1c averages of 8 or 9	Didn't change; felt guilty about it	I got other things under control that were causing the high averages	I changed over a dozen beliefs that lowered my HA1c results to the sixes
Blood Sugar tests frequently high	Guilt, futile attempts at self-discipline	I learned how to not hate testing	Hating to test was one of the first beliefs I changed
Infrequent testing	Recrimination, more attempts at will power	I learned how to not hate diabetes	I understood hating my disease was one of my biggest problems

My Problem	My Broken Old System	My Authentic Code	Note
Low energy	Nothing I tried worked	I increased my energy through exercise and lowering blood sugar levels	I became important to myself
High blood sugar upon waking	Couldn't solve without middle-of-the-night lows	I changed my belief to "My morning blood sugars are always in the target range"	Morning blood sugar readings are on target when I trust my intuition
Blood sugar fluctuations; spikes and severe lows	I tried the Insulin Pump but found I could not use it	I found an iPhone app that tracks my blood sugar and eliminates spikes and severe lows	I am off the pump but I recommend insulin pump therapy if it's right for you.
Embarrassed about diabetes; feeling inferior	Conscious effort to be more relaxed about diabetes	I became authentic about diabetes	
Angry at God and asking why	Better acceptance but it still nagged at me	I finally understood the *higher* education	Diabetes has been my greatest teacher

My Problem	My Broken Old System	My Authentic Code	Note
Lazy about taking care of it	I told myself I had good control and I was fine	I changed my belief that I'm lazy to "I want to take care of my body"	More help from above
I hated having diabetes	I put off testing because it reminded me how much I hated having diabetes	I decided to believe instead that *Diabetes is not a problem.*	Deciding to not hate something makes it so it doesn't come with a feeling attached.
I did not truly love myself	I was gradually doing better	I changed my beliefs about how I want to feel about myself	I had stopped this process before I was finished learning to truly love myself. I truly love myself now.
Diet high in simple carbohydrates	Reduced processed carbohydrates	I opened up to new ways and found solutions to the diet problem	I created a new structure for eating

Many of my problems are universal. If you don't have some of them, feel fortunate. If you don't have them you may have had them once and worked through them. But you have your own issues that trouble you and your code will evolve as mine has. As with everything, you will get better with practice. Now start to create your list.

Surround Yourself with a Support Team

I said in the beginning that this process is going to be simple but not easy. By now you can see why. In fact, you may be resisting like crazy. I know. I resisted too. The very best advice for this is to not try to do it alone. Get support. If you try it on your own your chance of giving up will be high. You will break your promise to yourself. You will begin to doubt you can do it. You'll decide I'm wrong. In fact, your resistance will become so strong you will stop. Remember – there are unseen forces at work that fight against our success!

It's like you're a rocket blasting off from Earth. Because of gravitational pull a rocket needs a huge quantity of fuel just to make the first few thousand feet into the air. But as it increases in altitude, as the atmosphere thins, it requires less and less energy until finally it reaches orbit where it can circle the earth indefinitely, using only tiny amounts of fuel to navigate into the proper position and stay on track.

That's a feeling you can look forward to, but I always tell people to expect the first breakthrough to take the largest amount of energy. Expect it to take the greatest amount time as well. My first big breakthrough essentially took twenty years, largely due to a severe stubborn streak and a limiting belief that techniques untried by me do not work. My second big breakthrough took about three months by comparison. I have been able to bring down the time it takes for a breakthrough to weeks and even days. And I occasionally have huge breakthroughs in just a few minutes.

It doesn't need to take twenty years, but if you're trying to do it alone you can bet discouragement will stop you. You need positive people in your life to encourage you, cheer you on, and tell you, *you can do it*. You can.

Some people don't have very supportive people in their lives. You may think they're supportive when in fact you are the one supporting them. You're going to have to test it. Just think about whether or not the person is your coach or your critic. That will make it clear. They may be supportive in other ways, just not in this way. You specifically need them to support your fragile new commitment to yourself. If they have never made such a commitment to themselves they may not be a good coach for you in this process.

If you find you don't have anyone, find someone. This is the first hurdle and where most people give up. It seems too hard for many people to make an effort to find their support team. Most people give up; most people feel moments of clarity once in a while, and then return to their original state of low energy and confusion.

Few people undertake to give it a one-hundred-per-cent-no-matter-what effort. And that's what it takes because it's hard at first – a practical no-matter-what approach. But trust me; it's only that difficult at first, and plenty of people besides me, many positive, supportive people, know it's worth every drop of sweat.

My favorite places for diabetes support are diabetes forums. There are many of them, some visited much more frequently than others. I go to diabeticconnect.com and I also visit diabetessisters.org. But it doesn't have to be online; anywhere you can find support, find it. I can't say it loud enough – *don't do this alone*. The risk of failure is just too high. You'll stop. I can promise that. But if you do stop, get started again, equipped with new knowledge of what you will have to do differently to succeed.

Deciding to make a commitment to change will show you where things stand when it comes to how you really feel. All sorts of objections will surface. Be ready for them and be ready to track them in a journal. Objections help strengthen your resolve. You need to be strong enough to blast off in those first few hundred feet or you will fall crashing to the ground.

What is Your Achilles Heel?

What keeps you from succeeding? Start developing a list of your troubles, along with ideas for how to overcome them. Go beneath the surface as best you can. You will be creating your plan using worksheets designed to drill down into your issues, but don't wait. Start right now. Understanding your core motivators, discussed earlier in this chapter, can help you. What seams easy? What's difficult?

I had a cavalier approach to diabetes that sabotaged my health for years. For a number of reasons I didn't want tight control, even though I knew poor control wasn't a good philosophy for long life; and my doctors, my family members, and my friends knew it too, and worried about me. When I finally began drilling beneath that issue I uncovered several big problems I had not been aware of. I didn't like myself. I was angry at God. I told myself I didn't even believe in God but really I was very, very ticked off! That was my Achilles heel. And how could God love me if He let this happen? So you can see why in my mind God did not think much of me. In my mind I was not important to God. My anger at God was beneath the surface.

Try to identify one major belief or behavior you know needs changing before anything else can change. What one thing would be huge for you if you could just change it? Refer to my chart for ideas about what you need to change. One clue is any negative emotion you feel when you think about things you don't like about yourself. Another clue to the big problem is *what do you not want it to be?* We will go into more detail about this later, so don't worry if you don't yet know what to work on first.

My startling revelation

Almost immediately upon finding awareness of my spiritual issues my authentic code appeared! My process makes diabetes feel like it's no big deal. Having diabetes is easy, it doesn't rob my energy, and it does not take away one bit from the quality of my life. That means

I'm in orbit. And once you are in orbit you feel as though you weigh next to nothing.

You will like being in orbit too, with only tiny bits of fuel needed to keep you in your proper position. Being in orbit means you will be moving forward with a tremendous amount of energy toward your next big adventure, whatever that may be.

Part 2. The Four Ways You Use Energy

Chapter 3. Energy: The Foundation of Health

Your Energy Core

My code came to me spelled out in four energy *languages* that helped me understand myself and the world. It became very clear to me once I understood myself and identified my unique diabetes code, that everything is about your energy. Our personalities can essentially be reduced to what motivates us – what energizes us. Whether or not you are doing what you want to be doing with your life and whether or not you behave in ways that serve you, it's all based on energy. Before we dive into these four facets, though, I want to look more closely at energy itself; when it is low you want to know why it's low and what you can do to increase it.

Experts in self-development and behavior modification agree that the first step in bringing change to an issue is awareness that change is needed. There are two things to understand when you don't feel good; 1) You need change, and 2) Your energy is probably low, making change difficult. Most people's energy is so low they know they need to change something but they don't change. Sound familiar? Low energy is why it took so long for me to begin to change. But my energy rose higher and higher as I got better at raising it.

My favorite resource on energy is *The Power of Full Engagement*, by sports psychologists Jim Loehr and Tony Schwartz (Loehr and Schwartz, 2003). Their work helped me to understand energy, though the word *energy* had baffled me for a long time before picking up the book; when people said my energy was low I was confused by it and I didn't know how to increase it. Then I cracked my own energy code! Once you begin to understand, you will know what I'm talking a about.

There are only four sources of energy in the human body. Once you use up all your energy you are done until you sleep, rest, or at least, do something you love to do. Exercise will give you energy to do more in less time than you spend exercising. There are foods that increase energy and foods that decrease energy. Following is a brief overview of energy and what you are doing to increase and decrease it in four very unique ways.

You can physically deplete energy, as you can deplete it with the other three sources, but physical energy is the only energy source we deliberately renew. Physical sources of energy include eating, relaxing, sleeping, and exercise. As I mentioned before, sleep restores energy, as does rest and relaxation. You can become rejuvenated by meditating, taking a nap, actively working at something you love, or by simply sitting quietly. Vacations renew enough energy to help for a month or more (of course if you don't spend enough time relaxing on vacation you may come home more tired than when you left). To keep from becoming burned out you must include enough sleep and free time every day. You can count as free time anything you do for your soul, that is, anything you do because you love doing it.

I could write a volume on how different foods affect energy, both to increase and to decrease it. I will devote more time to the discussion of foods in Chapter 4.

The body is the manifestation of the soul. Some things we crave are soulful desires. But we are conditioned in our society to deny our body's needs and not to give in to its so-called temptations. This is a mistake as these desires will necessarily come out, whether in ways within your control or in darker ways as cravings and even addictions. So include activities in your day that are good for your soul. Even my healthcare practitioners suggest that one cookie or glass of wine will not send my blood sugar spiraling or plummeting – it's when I deprive myself of these things that problems with over-indulgence arise.

We use mental energy by focusing and concentrating on tasks: thinking, writing, reading, working at the computer, and even driving, require and expend mental energy. Obsessive/compulsive and impulse behaviors use a lot of mental energy. If you have these types of behaviors please seek professional help. Decreasing negative behaviors will increase your energy, besides helping in other ways. The higher your energy is the easier it will be to stay in control and the happier you will be.

You may be wondering what I mean by emotional energy. Like everything in the universe, emotions are vibrations. The lowest emotions vibrate at a very low frequency, like the low notes on a piano keyboard. Which emotions feel lowest to you? I think apathy is the very lowest. People with depression are often apathetic. At the opposite end of the keyboard are the highest notes; they vibrate at such a high level they look like a straight line on paper. Their emotional equivalents are feelings like acceptance and love. At times you can feel so light it isn't even a feeling. It's more a state of being. We will talk more about this emotionally charged topic further into the book.

The unconscious use of spiritual energy is the biggest energy zapper by far. But how can you avoid using up spiritual energy?

First and most obvious, love yourself. I was unintentionally taught to not love myself and I find that the majority of people are unconsciously taught this too. You love your wife, your husband, your children, and your parents, but are you aware of whether or not you love yourself *just as much*? Are you afraid loving yourself is self-centered?

You may love even your pets more than you love yourself. This one-sided kind of love is a silly double standard though. Why would _____ (your higher power, God, the universe) say you should love everybody but yourself? Are you somehow not as important as someone else? Anybody else? Do you see how preposterous it sounds when I put it that way? Let it be OK to love yourself.

If you're not sure just admit that you don't love yourself. Why would I say that? Because people who love themselves know they do. If you don't love yourself begin to love yourself. Everything else, including your relationship with your higher power, your relationships with the people you love, and your sense of why you're here, hinges on your ability to love yourself. And it's the cornerstone of energy.

Figure out your relationship with your higher power. What on Earth are you here to do? I look at the expenditure of spiritual energy like trying to find some place when you don't have the address, you don't know the area, and you don't know in which direction to go. You would use a lot of gas driving around *hoping* to get lucky.

Most of us are unbalanced in several ways, whether you are happy or unhappy in your marriage, your job, or your life. Unhealthiness in any of the four ways you use energy will bring your energy low because you will not be meeting your energy needs. We all need refueling. But it's mostly by increasing your spiritual energy that you will find the strength you need to change. Learning about the types of energy and how you expend it can help you conserve it for use in ways you choose. Through the four sources of energy you will find the exact combination that comprises your code – the system you will use to live a happy, fulfilling, and useful life with or without diabetes.

The features of physical and mental energy

Chances are you weren't eating and exercising in ways that benefitted you before you got diabetes. Suddenly you are ordered to do things you always knew you did not want to do. This makes the journey to physical healthiness a grueling one. It begins with taking responsibility.

Face it: weight loss, balance, a healthy lifestyle, and cutting out sugar, processed carbohydrates, soft drinks, and alcohol may be changes you know you ought to make but instead avoid making. Asking yourself a few pointed questions can help you begin the process of unraveling what you are doing and not doing to support your body and your future.

Your body is the most meaningful expression of your soul. That means if you don't like your body you don't like yourself and you are disconnected from your very soul. So how much do you like your body?

How does the idea that *you have created it to be the way it is* make you feel? Feelings create behaviors. How you feel about something creates the results you get. Remember, every step you take in the direction you want to go gets you closer to your goal. Simply realizing you are depressed or acknowledging an eating disorder is good. It's telling you the direction you must go, though it will be up to you to get there.

Before I was diagnosed with diabetes I was at my ideal weight. I didn't over-do sweets or eat a lot of junk food. I got some exercise, but even now I can do better when it comes to exercise. We were planning our second child when I suddenly developed Type 1 diabetes.

My doctor told me I must wait at least six months before becoming pregnant. I had to go through a "honeymoon" with my disease, he told me. I needed to get familiar with it. I'm not very systematic and I didn't want to have diabetes (who does?), so I wasn't very good at following my doctor's advice. The extent of my system was to wait the six months and then decide it was OK to get pregnant.

Then I had a miscarriage. It was a big wake-up call about the seriousness of my situation. I had already heard about horror stories of spinal bifida and other health problems of babies born in diabetes type pregnancies. I began to realize that if I did not take control of my disease I had no right to bring another human being into the world.

So when I became pregnant again I went through my pregnancy with a team of specialists to guide me. I saw a special doctor and got my

HA1c levels down to the sixes before even starting. I learned all I could about pregnancy and diabetes and took it to heart. I was a model of obedience and conformity; I reported my tracking to my nurse every day, including every morsel I ate, every gram of carbohydrate, protein, and fat. I reported each of my 10-12 daily glucose readings. I adhered strictly to the diet high in protein, complex carbohydrates, and rich nutrients, and devoid of sugar. My nurse reported the results to my doctor and the team monitored and adjusted my insulin doses as my pregnancy progressed. It was a great system and since I had lots of coaches my baby girl was perfect – healthy and beautiful.

My experience with pregnancy showed me I could do it. But after my daughter was born I began a period of uncontrolled binge eating. I ate sugary junk food until I felt sick. I didn't want to test because I already knew the results were high. I was guilty, depressed, angry, alone, and DIS-eased; completely out of control of my illness. I was so ashamed I did not want to find people to help me. What I experienced was a complete reversal of what I had been able to do when I was pregnant.

I had the classic symptoms of an eating disorder. The result over the next several months was HA1c results of eleven and twelve. I slowly and gradually gained control over my numbers but I will always remember how strange it was that I never had any kind of problem with eating until I had diabetes. Having diabetes magnified my other problems and brought new ones I didn't have before.

Something else occurred to me. While I was pregnant I was able to do all the right things for this other person growing inside me, but once she was born it was like the dam broke. I could not do the same for myself. And as it dawned on me that my thinking was wrong I began to understand that since my daughter and I are both human beings we should be equally valuable and precious. Right? It was exactly the catalyst for change I needed.

Before developing diseases like diabetes, heart disease, digestive ailments, cancer, and other major illnesses, people almost always have other health issues they weren't previously paying attention to and they were certainly not aware of the effect their health was having on their performance and the quality of their lives. This was true for me and it's true for most of the people I work with.

Underlying every physical symptom people with diabetes experience there lies a mental DIS-ease. When you start to uncover the underlying causes of obesity, unhealthy eating, unhealthy lifestyle choices, and failure to create healthy alternatives you will probably find that your mental processes are creating your unwanted results. That's why I insist that people look seriously at what is going on in their minds and bring it all to the light. Without light on the problem people must rely solely on will-power.

The will-power myth

I believe will-power is a poor approach to bringing about change for most people. Many experts will back me up because people do what we are programmed to do unless we consciously change the programming. If will-power alone could have changed the course of my life I probably would not have diabetes. I could not and you will not either. This isn't bad news, but you have some work ahead to change your programming.

Your doctor, dietitian, and other professionals have given you instructions for physical care. You probably own several books and subscribe to periodicals. There are seminars and classes. The education has been right in front of you but once you have begun to change your programming you will have more of a desire to pay attention to it. The education you have received about how to live a healthy lifestyle will have fertile ground on which to take root.

Making healthier changes led me to become more open to learning about diet: pH balance, the value of a nutritional fat-based-low-carb diet, simple vs. complex carbohydrates, and how complex carbohydrates create higher energy and lessen binge-eating because of the slower and more consistent release of sugar into the body. Who knew that foods in their whole form have fewer carbohydrates while being more filling, and that replacing carbs with the proper fats (Omega-3, not vegetable fat) can actually help me lose weight? I didn't pay attention when I didn't care so much about taking care of my body.

Having the right pH balance will boost your immune system. Exercise helps you lose weight, gives you energy, and benefits your immune system. Getting the proper amount of sleep, rest, and relaxation gives you more energy. You can also increase energy by doing things that bring you pleasure.

I became open to learning more about insulin; how dosing insulin differs from the effects of healthy peoples' naturally occurring insulin and how fat positively affects blood sugar due to slower metabolism. I know why when I eat pizza and Chinese food I can have lows an hour or two later, then spikes of high blood sugar four or more hours after eating it. And I know what I can do so I can still enjoy the occasional pizza.

Metabolism varies from person to person. As time goes on, you will learn more about your body and will be able to find physical solutions to help you live the lifestyle you want, whether it's enjoying the occasional dessert, or participating in a sport you love. You will find you still have a life and there is nothing to stop you from living it.

And without self-love, simply having a healthy knowledge about diet, understanding energy, and lowering your stress levels would matter little because you would not care. Begin to get healthy-minded by confronting your DIS-ease; then get to know your body and you will be surprised at how easy and even how much fun loving your body can be.

Commitments to yourself

To find power that will actually help you, let's look at something that does not use will-power. It requires self-love. It's the notion of keeping commitments you make to yourself. If you make a promise to yourself and you do not keep it you will have a harder time keeping the next one. You let yourself off the hook each time you do not honor the commitment you made, making it easier and easier to break promises you make to yourself until *you can no longer believe a word you say*. Keeping the agreements you make with yourself and others increases your confidence. Not keeping them erodes your confidence.

Emotional and Mental Wellness

Every thought comes with a feeling, or how you feel about the thought. Emotions are the fuel that drives action. But heavy emotions can weigh you down. Did you know that you can simply release what is weighing you down and feel more energetic? That you can pinpoint what weighs you down and keeps you from feeling like yourself? For me it was anger. Most people with diabetes tell me that anger affects their diabetes control. I was angry about having diabetes for many years and I definitely had poor control as a result.

My father had diabetes and at the age of thirty I developed it. The diagnosis completely derailed me. My life felt *over*. I fell under the diabetes shadow; gloomy, depressed, and angry. And my father didn't help; "It's easy to deal with. It's no big deal," he said many times before he succumbed to kidney failure. That *he* was the focus of much of my anger didn't help (we'll discuss forgiveness later).

Over the next two decades I didn't realize I was outraged at my father, myself, and God. If there were times I realized my outrage I ignored them. I thought there was nothing I could do about it and that thought overwhelmed me. I believed that there was not one good thing about having diabetes.

Is the term *Happy Diabetic* an oxymoron? Not when you understand mental states – specifically how a positive attitude affects your health when it comes to treating diabetes. Dark emotions are at the core of most diseases. They carry a message you can either choose to listen to or choose not to. I finally listened to it. It said, "Let go of your pain." Are you holding onto anger at a disease? Are you trying to ignore it? Instead, you could try acknowledging it and giving your anger at the disease the attention it demands – as though it was an injured child. When you face anger in this way its power over you diminishes. And in its place comes gradual peace.

Seven practical reasons why your emotions affect your control

My diabetes care providers focus on the physical aspects of diabetes control and do not dive into the deeper issues of how emotional and mental states of mind contribute to poor diabetes control, even though being in a negative emotional state hinders control. While many people with diabetes acknowledge they know what to do, too often there is a big gap between knowing it and doing it. This is where the mind comes in. Keep in mind these seven points about emotional and mental diabetes control.

1. Self-sabotage. If you are not aware of how you sabotage yourself you will keep doing it. As Einstein said, "A problem can never be solved at the level at which it was created." Becoming aware brings it to the new level needed for change. The first thing to do to change behavior is to become aware of the behavior that you need to change.

2. Same old pattern. New behaviors require a conscious shift in thinking and then taking action on the new belief. But conversely, taking action can help you develop new healthier attitudes and beliefs; it works both ways. If you are having trouble changing an old undesirable belief, try a new behavior that reinforces the new belief. We have a method you can use to change beliefs instantly, which we will discuss in a later chapter.

3. Habit. Deliberate actions repeated over time will help develop new habits. If you have tried in vain to develop new habits, try this; don't change everything at once. Choose one new habit, practice it until it becomes natural, and then move to the next one. Changing one habit increases your habit-changing skills, too. You'll be surprised at how much quicker and easier your progress becomes.

4. No system. For methodical people a good system will be quite easy and will only require small adjustments to refine what you are already doing. For everyone else, to keep from getting too frustrated you'll need to develop a blueprint that's ideal for you; so get help. This book will help you do it.

5. Emotional choosing. Regardless of how disciplined you are you may be unaware that you are making emotional decisions that adversely affect your diet and diabetes control, rather than rational decisions of your conscious choosing that affect you positively.

6. Stress. Your stress level and mental state of mind cause behaviors you may regret later, piling on guilt.

7. Experiences. Remembering past experiences and feeling the emotions that come with them may be affecting your behaviors negatively without you even knowing it.

Take your temperature

It's important to understand and deal with your emotions when trying to control diabetes. If you are unhappy with your level of diabetes control, what is your emotional state of mind and what aspects of it are affecting your glucose levels? Start by thinking of one obvious one.

Do you want to be more youthful and fun, even though you happen to have the symptom of diabetes? Start by taking your current emotional temperature. Did you know that a part of you, your authentic self, is already healthy and happy? If that's not how you know you feel, you have work to do.

There are several ways to be energetic and happily living your life, not in spite of your disease, but in sync with it. Rule Number One:

don't swim against the current. That's my definition of stress. Learn to let go of what you're holding on to. By lowering the stress caused by a heavy work load, not enough *me* time, and the demands of a family, you will let go of some of the heavy emotions that are causing you to feel sluggish.

I don't mean to suggest that it will be easy. You are turning around beliefs and behaviors that you have been comfortable with for a long time, regardless of how unhappy you are believing them. Ours is a culture of negativity so for most of us pessimism feels normal. That's because emotions are pure energy and as energy they have weight – in the form of wavelengths. The darker emotions have long waves or vibrations, and the lighter the emotion the shorter the wave length. And it's easier to go over to the negative. Positive emotions are pure; the most pure emotion is peace, and its vibration is so high it's almost impossible to detect the feeling; it's more of a state of being. The lowest emotions, the ones that feel the strongest, have a lower vibration and are easier to detect. These vibrations include dread, fear, and apathy.

We discussed how in musical terms low notes have low frequencies and the higher the note the higher the frequency. Emotionally speaking, higher frequencies are more challenging and much less comfortable to sustain. This is why people stay in a low energy state; we tend to do what is easiest – especially those of us living with illnesses like diabetes. That's why I will always tell you to start with the one thing that, if you could succeed at it, would really change your life and help you change everything else you want to change.

How about something you can do right now?

Hold on to your emotions and you will continue to re-live the stress they cause. You're simply remembering the anger, or fear, or confusion you felt a moment before. Emotions aren't long lasting, they're fleeting. You feel it one moment, and the next moment you feel something else. But acknowledge your emotion of the moment and it will simply vanish. This method is great to use with unpleasant feelings.

For the nice ones, go ahead and hold onto them, and the memory of them, for as long as you possibly can.

Goals

Of course everyone wants the best possible life, but this seems like a lot of work! It will be worth it because with goals that you make and keep, you can expect to feel great all of the time. You will be the happiest you have ever been! Happier even than before you developed diabetes. And you will find it becomes very easy to stay in great control. Your doctor will pat you on the back and wonder what changed. There is no down side.

As you know, the healthiest and happiest people have healthy minds. The process is simple but, at least at first, not easy, since mastery can only come with strong commitment and lots of practice.

Take a moment to be honest with yourself; are you healthy minded and positive? All the time? If not, what would it take to get you to that level? A good goal will give you a healthier mental state, not sporadically but regularly. Your new goal could be yoga; learning to meditate or visualize; learning how to let go; focusing on gratitude; or nurturing your soul in a meaningful way. Anything you have wanted to begin doing and have not been successful will be a good goal to start with.

Let's choose a goal or new habit of gratitude as an example. Gratitude, it has been proven, lowers blood pressure and releases calming endorphins into the blood. Have you ever noticed that when you switch from the negative to having gratitude your perspective shifts? You feel lighter, calmer, and better able to proceed.

As part of your strategy you will want to list things you can do that will make you feel grateful. Choose at least three actions to do each day. They can be the same each day or different, you decide. And you will want to set a deadline.

It takes twenty-one days to develop a new habit. Give yourself 30 days to get into the habit, in case you backslide. Feeling the benefits of a habit is the easiest way to keep it, so choose things that will make you feel happy. After the habit is formed you must continue to practice and make choices in favor of the habit, although it won't require as much conscious thinking over time.

What are the best ways to get started then? Writing daily in a gratitude journal is an easy way to develop a positive attitude. You can choose to write a specific number of things you are grateful for, like three things each day, or you can keep it close and write in it throughout the day as you feel inspired. Remember, one aspect of this as a goal is caring about you, so don't forget to have gratitude for your own insights and accomplishments.

Search the Internet for gratitude; websites where you can make contributions and benefit from another's gratitude. Send a thank-you-note-a-day to the people who make you happy. Whatever you do, make sure it's fun. If you are thinking this exercise sounds silly, remember, it's the discomfort of it that is so powerful. Again, this is about what's best for you, no one else. Remember that although it seems trivial, a little gratitude goes a long way. Having gratitude is a very effective and powerful way to become more positive naturally.

Is there something you love to do that you're not doing? Is it spending time with people who are like you? Hugging your cat? Inviting friends for dinner? Civil War re-enactments? These are soulful activities. If you know what you love to do, do more of it. If you don't know what you love to do, find out. Then do more of it.

Everything rewarding is challenging because for every action there is an equal and opposite reaction. For every new level of joy you want there will be a level of difficulty and challenge to reach it. If you want to truly change do not stop your forward direction. It will delay your progress and your success. And do not give up because you are not seeing change. This process requires time and patience, two things we don't seem to have a lot of in our society. Going deep requires slowing down. And going deep is the idea.

So your progress isn't apparent. What then? It's like you have to take two steps forward and one step back. Remember, you are human, there is a lot to learn, and we are our own worst enemies when it comes to growing and changing. Remember that even though you don't see progress, it's there; it just takes more time than you think. Whenever someone asks me how long it will take to start to see results I always say, "Longer than you want it to. I can guarantee that." But we don't want it to take a long time. We live in a world of instant gratification and if we don't begin to see results immediately we often conclude that the idea did not work. That's what I did for a long time.

A more positive way to see progress will be to look back three or six months ago to see what you have done. And you will really be able to see progress when you get to where you cannot even imagine going back. That's a breakthrough. You wouldn't be able to go back to your old thinking even if you tried. Nobody who makes these changes in his or her life ever goes back. That's how you know it's true, authentic, right, and important.

Don't Be Negative, Sick, and Ineffective

I mentioned at the beginning of this chapter that there are forces working to make you ineffective. Before we move on we need to talk more about this idea. Whether the voices come from within you or outside of you (a matter of personal belief), this much I know for sure: my inner talk was making me weak and ineffective and it was killing me. Unless you are aware of it, it's probably killing you too.

For me, religion did not stop the voices. Religious principles I subscribed to did not seem to acknowledge the criticisms that played endlessly in my head day and night. And the voices are not just in *my* head; many, many people I know tell me about the internal accusations and criticism they are forced to listen to. We get so accustomed to the constant blaming that eventually we don't even hear it – until it becomes VERY LOUD. In case you're still not sure what I'm talking about think about the last time you wanted to curl up on the sofa and read a good book. If I do this I will soon hear a voice telling me to get my work done first. It keeps me from being able to enjoy the book and if I agree with it I'll stop reading and go back to my tasks.

Think about how you felt the last time someone told you, "You look really nice today." The voice in your head might say, "He's just hitting on you," or "She's just saying that to make you feel better," or my favorite, "That's not true because I know I look awful." The response you give to that person may even be *exactly what the voice just told you* – the thing you believe.

These are examples of one force in nature that's at work to bring you down and it works if you believe it. Where do the voices come from? Most psychologists say they are memories of things you were told a long time ago. Children are extremely impressionable, and remember, human memory is so good that humans are the only "animals" that punish themselves and one another repeatedly for a single mistake.

Many spiritual and religious groups attribute the voices to spirit entities outside ourselves – like the image of the devil and angel sitting atop one's shoulders, whispering opposing advice into each ear, and making judgments when you decide what to do. Regardless of your personal philosophy or theology about where the voices come from, we cannot deny they exist.

The voices are why I took twenty years to learn to love myself. From the day I first found out it was possible to learn to love myself those voices became louder and more insistent, practically driving me crazy with, "You're nothing. You'll never change. You're unlikeable. You're not good enough." They effectively slowed, and at times stopped my progress altogether. I still hear the voices to this day. The difference is now I recognize them as destroyers of my health, happiness, and fulfillment in life and they don't have power over me unless I agree with them.

This is spiritual combat, depleting energy on a spiritual level. It's literally killing us. I've blogged a lot over the years about diabetes and one comment I hear more than anything else is, "I know what to do but I just don't do it." Why would a person choose not to do the things that would give them energy today, and life and health far out into the future? It's the voices.

How do you get rid of the voices? You can't; anyone who tells you that you can is listening to voices. In a typical day we have approximately 80,000 thoughts. And each thought comes with its corresponding feeling. For most people about three-fourths of them are undesirable. For most of my life the majority of my thoughts were negative judgments about me, my body, God, other people, and my circumstances. Most of the time I was not even aware of them, but they would zap my energy nonetheless. When I was aware of them they seemed to zap my energy even more. I actually believed I was powerless to do anything about the feelings they prompted. So *I know what to do but I'm just not doing it,* was typical thinking for me.

This spiritual energy drain is the reason we live lives chained to a disease. It zaps more energy than physical, mental, and emotional factors combined. It's a vicious downward spiral, like water flushing down a drain. The biggest lie ever perpetrated on the human race has been, "There's nothing you can do about it."

Don't listen to that for one more second.

Years ago I had a mentor who was a Christian Minister. He taught me how to love myself, and that it was good, not bad (some religions teach that self-love is a sin, as my former religion had done). I had lived more than thirty years believing that I was unlovable and too broken to fix; that I should just give up. Imagine living with that belief every single day. It is a wonder I survived thirty years, though plenty of other miserable people have not survived it.

Even though my mentor worked with me for three years on how to love myself, and even though I enjoyed some amazing breakthroughs and my life became much better, I still wasn't healthy. See, I thought I was better; I thought I was done and free to go on with my life. I thought

I was whole. But I still had angry outbursts and I still *suffered* with diabetes. It would take another twenty years to work through it all.

I was still mad at God, justifiably, and I didn't even know it. I decided I didn't know or care whether I still believed or not. I was as focused on myself as ever, and I still hated taking care of diabetes. I was a little less difficult to be with. I made some strides in those years; I got a college degree, I survived being fired, I moved into a better career, and I got a Master's degree – all in that twenty years. I understood the concept of loving myself and at times I was able to, but from beneath my personal surface, doubt, fear, and mediocrity bubbled up – ineffective, destructive mediocrity. What I really wanted was to be free. And what I thought was that it was impossible because, "How could I be free from Type 1 Diabetes, when my insulin producing cells died years ago?"

When I received my master's degree I knew I was ready for something better. I wanted a fulfilling career I could throw myself into completely; not just a job. When it happened I had to pinch myself to make sure it was real. I had applied for, and was offered, a position as a personal coach for clients of Success Coach Jack Canfield, whose name is synonymous with Chicken Soup. I was a coach of *The Success Principles* program based on his book by the same name (Canfield, 2005).

As a mentor I learned to teach people about beliefs, negative programming, releasing their brakes, affirmations, visualizing, self-esteem, and goals. I quickly fell into the rhythm of coaching and my self-esteem shot up as I found I was good at it. I knew I was good because people's lives changed. What it did for me was even bigger – it held me accountable.

I was living my dream and working in my dream job when I soon realized that if a person is in alignment with what they are meant to do, a job can fun, easy, and doesn't feel one bit like work. But once I began advising other people to face their fears and push through them I realized something even greater. I had three fingers pointing back at me. I'm no hypocrite so it was time for me to step up.

I began by changing my dark inner talk, something I had not believed possible before because nothing I had tried had ever worked. I committed to working only on my self-talk. I used positive affirmations religiously, and I made a commitment not to try to change everything at once. This was intuitive, something I only realized later. It took less than two months to go from being a negative person to being positive most of the time. And once you do it your life will become much, much easier.

I paid attention to the incessant accusations coming from my own mind. I had not realized how frequent, how loud, and how effective they were at stopping me and rendering my whole life a useless waste. Wow! Life soon felt overwhelming as the voices seemed to get louder and more insistent. Once I paid attention to them it was as though they were holding on for dear life. I actually give my voices names; as I mentioned, some people believe the voices are spiritual entities literally doing battle on a spiritual plane.

After about two months of working steadily on my inner talk and feeling I was making some progress, I woke up one morning feeling very warm and happy. I'd had an incredible night's sleep. I was awake, alert, and energized. What was different about this morning compared to other mornings? Then it occurred to me. For the first time ever, I think, I felt positive when I woke up.

I'm not a morning person, but for the first time I had energy and didn't feel cranky. I felt happy for no logical reason. Not a fleeting sort of happiness like random happiness I had felt from time to time. This felt very different. This feeling was permanent.

"What was different?" I wondered.

Well, I had this incredible dream where I had been in charge of some massive operation. I was standing in the middle of the area on a platform and countless people came up to me to ask what they should do about this or that important task. As I gave them advice and direction they were grateful I was there to help them solve their problems. I understood that we were doing something significant and I was at the center of it, orchestrating it as though I had been born to lead. When I woke up it occurred to me that I had never before had such a powerful dream, where I was in charge and everything was working. In my dreams I had always been running scared or naked – situations that had always left me feeling embarrassed and victimized. I had never before been in control in a dream.

What was different? I was different. I was transformed. All I could think was, "Oh my God!" It was true. It had really happened to me. I was, as they said in my former religion, *born again*, although then I had not experienced it like this. So this was what it felt like.

The most important energy source

Believe in yourself and you will gain everything else worth having. If you believe in yourself you will love your fellow man. You will be a great parent, child, wife, husband, lover, and friend. You will love God and feel loved by and important to God. Your greatest source of energy is belief in yourself.

As I progressed from becoming a person newly in love with myself other opportunities for learning began to appear. My ego, which I call the low self, was in charge for more than fifty years and I am still sorting out how to keep my authentic self at the helm as much as possible. But my highest self mostly runs the show.

We are each here for of some divine reason. Most of us spend our lives just trying to sort that out. Since I am now divinely connected to what is true and right I have found meaning in my life. And I know that bringing my code to people suffering with diabetes as I was is part of it. This is my great source of infinite energy.

Principles for starting

My system was broken, I did not know it was broken, and I believed living with diabetes was always going to be hard. But once I fixed what was broken spiritually the rest fell into place for me. That is my particular path; yours may be similar or it could be quite different. Regardless, these principles will help you when you have trouble.

You will find resistance to the ideas here and for some it will even cause you to stop. I've mentioned this before and it bears repeating. If you find you have slowed way down or even stopped working don't add insult to injury by criticizing yourself. It's natural to stop. We've talked about the many reasons it happens. Now I want to lay down a few guidelines for reference when you have trouble.

1. *Try different solutions*. You may need to try a few different techniques to find what works for you. It's OK. You won't know until you try it. I have bought shoes because I liked them only to find they weren't right. Some shoes I know immediately are not right; they look wonderful until I put them on. I also have shoes that have been my favorites for years.

Give yourself permission to try on an idea; if the idea doesn't work you have lost a little but you have gained valuable knowledge and you can put that one out of your mind and move on. I have spent time and money trying on different ideas. I approach it as education because without those chances I took that weren't what I wanted I wouldn't be where I am now. Decide just to try it on. You may need to invest a little. It will be worth the risk. But don't decide too soon that it doesn't work. Personal growth strategies, unlike buying shoes, take longer to "try on."

2. *Be completely honest with yourself*. Be more honest with yourself than you are with anyone else. Be more honest with yourself than you are with God. This is the highest level of maturity and it takes a lot of courage. But ninety per cent of what you aren't being honest about is directed at you *by* you. For some reason we don't believe that we need to hold ourselves to the very highest level of accountability.

Or maybe that's an excuse. If you are in this category it is hurting your self-esteem more and more each time you do it. Consider how much of the time you don't tell the truth to yourself. Keeping your agreements with other people is not the problem; it's keeping your agreements to yourself. Having integrity to yourself must come first. Do everything as though someone else is watching. Someone is – your high self.

3. *You need energy*. You need enough energy to fly on your own power. In the movie *The Flight of the Phoenix* the men needed enough speed and momentum to fly off the cliff and not crash at the bottom. At first it's hard to start the climb up out of the fall. It takes all the energy and dedication you can muster.

4. *It takes time*. Over time you will find you begin to feel a rhythm. At first it will feel like an awakening. Then you will notice a breakthrough in your thinking. Things start to become easier. Your energy increases. Then one day you realize you've changed and you will never go back to the old you.

5. *Examine your beliefs*. Beliefs are very powerful but you can change them. I had to concentrate on my first belief changes and consciously take action to support them, a physical activity. For example, you may think you don't deserve to have some item you want. One way to help change that belief is to surprise yourself by buying it.

   If buying the thing makes you feel guilty, the guilt may just be coming from a belief that you don't deserve to have what you want. A thought comes to you that you're not supposed to want things for yourself – that it's selfish. You may have been raised to believe it was a fact, that you didn't need it or even deserve it, by people who didn't know they were teaching you this limiting belief. Interestingly enough, this same belief keeps them from deserving what they want too.

6. *Put yourself first with this project*. If selfishness feels wrong to you, you could be sabotaging your success by telling yourself that working on yourself is selfish. If something is deemed to be selfish to you, you will shy away from it, believing it tells the world that you are selfish. But there is a distinction. Selfishness is not related to self-nurturing and self-care at all. When your own nurturing needs aren't met you usually don't even know it. And if you believe everything you do for yourself is selfish you can bet your needs aren't met and you are unaware of it – unconsciously you don't know how to get nurtured. In truth, selfishness is fake whereas self-nurturing is real.

If you haven't been nurtured properly, how much do you think people receive from your empty pitcher? When I was full of DIS-ease my nurturing needs were not met. I wanted to give and help other people and every attempt was exhausting. It wasn't until I learned to meet my own needs that I realized I had been trying to pour from an empty pitcher. If you first fill up your pitcher you will be able to pour true nurturing from it to the people you want to help.

7. *Gather your support.* If your family does not support achievement of your goals you are likely a victim of negative and harmful programming. Not to place blame; it just means you have old beliefs that came from people who meant well but were themselves stuck. They may tell you that the life you dream of is impossible and your ideas and goals are not practical. They may say you are not capable of accomplishing them.

One woman told me when she was young she had great artistic ability. She wanted to be a professional illustrator. Her father said the field was too competitive, and worse, if she kept pursuing it he would not pay for her college. Her mother told her she is a follower not a leader, that she has a weak personality, and that she needed to be careful. When I met her twenty-five years later the words still echoed in her head telling her why she will always be ordinary.

8. *Clear out the bugs* *in your head.* Have you ever ridden a motorcycle? You have a nice big face shield on your helmet. You're cruising down the freeway at 65. You hit a bug storm and suddenly you can't see. You will have to exit and clean it before you can continue. All the doubts in your head from well-meaning people, themselves afraid to take big steps, are like bugs on your face shield. When those doubts come in remind yourself they are bugs on your belief window so you can clean them off and see clearly.

9. *Let go of the brakes*. It will take *the amount of time it takes you* to get out of your own way and break through to where you want to be. The time it takes is affected by fear; fear that you're not good enough, smart enough, or capable enough. Believing you can't do it is why you're not doing it. Understand what it is you are telling yourself causing you to believe you can't do it. As you become better at confronting what you are unhappy about each day it's like you are releasing the brakes on your life. You don't need to push on the gas, just let go of the brake to gain momentum and begin to move faster.

10. *Take time*. At first you may find yourself saying "I don't have time." If you take time anyway you will begin to see the value of the process after only a short while. When people say "I don't have time" they are really saying "I won't take the time." But if instead you put a higher value on the time you take for this process you will easily find the time to do it.

As I said earlier, only three per cent of people really take this journey. We tell ourselves it's not important when really it's just too scary. Not having time is actually an excuse not to look within, and the excuse is rooted in fear. This is the case with anything you have wanted to do for a long time and have never done.

11. *Make developing your authentic diabetes code a breakthrough goal*. The definition of a breakthrough goal is that it would require a breakthrough in your thinking to be able to accomplish it, and that in your current thinking you really do not believe you can do it. You are thinking negatively and the negativity will never get you to your goal. If you set the goal anyway, and if you stick with it, you will change your thinking, which will enable you to take a position you may never have seen yourself take before.

12. *Use Affirmations to directly reverse your damaging inner talk.* Hearing what you say to yourself is the key. An affirmation is a positive statement you make even though you don't believe it. Examples are, *I am brilliant, people really like me, I am a money magnet,* and *I am enough.* I devote an entire section on how to create your own affirmations in Chapter 8. Start by creating one right now.

Affirmations work because they say the opposite in a positive way. You are speaking directly to primary issues. Does it feel uncomfortable to you to read your affirmation? If not, do something that will make it feel uncomfortable, like saying it out loud in front of the mirror. Or saying it to your spouse. The discomfort of it is the key; if affirmations are flat and don't have meaning they will be weak. The feelings of awkwardness and discomfort are what make them powerful. The discomfort comes from not really believing it at some level.

Affirmations help you see the two parts of you; the side that believes and the side that doesn't. The more uncomfortable it is to say the opposite of what you believe the more good you are doing; there is a belief that you are not that person, but there is also deeper core knowledge that you *are* that person. You are calling up a deeper knowledge that you *can* do it and winning out over the part of you that says you can't.

13. *If you know you need help with self-esteem there are several good resources.* Jack Canfield's Maximum Confidence program targets low self-esteem (Canfield, 2002). Most of us grow up doubting ourselves. The real culprit is the discomfort of getting out of the habit of complacency. Most of what we have talked about in these principles is the result of your habits. Change your habits about how you feel about yourself and you will change your life.

14. *The authors of The Power of Full Engagement* (Loehr and Schwartz, 2003) recommend you *look at life more as a series of sprints and less as a marathon.* A sprinter goes fast, rests, and goes into the next meet where he sprints fast then rests again. He is able to go fast again because of the rest period. He knows he can give it everything in the short race because he knows exactly how long he needs to sustain the high speed.

15. *Are your* [bad] *choices mistakes or life lessons?* Our failures in life teach us much more than what we learn from our successes. These lessons help you in the future, even if the lesson seems unrelated. Perhaps you are learning it now while it is a minor mistake; if you learn it later it could be costlier – even deadly.

A man I know was married for five years before he realized it was a mistake. He talked often about the five years he had *wasted*. It was such a big deal to him that he *wasted* another two years trying to salvage the marriage – the five lost years. They were not wasted, he was just looking at it wrong, and his behavior reflected it.

Looking at an investment of time or money you have made can get in the way of the decision you need to make next. Often we think we can't survive our [bad] decisions but we can. Get it done and get on with your life, appreciating the value of what you learned; *knowing when to hold 'em, and when to fold 'em.* People who have survived unspeakable events and circumstances would never ask to go through it again, but many are still able to turn the experience around and make something positive from it. The level of *who we are* is much deeper than what happens to us. Nothing can hurt who you are at your core. Other people and life's experiences can only hurt your ego.

My clients have used the above principles for everything from overcoming debilitating shyness to becoming millionaires. I have used them to conquer diabetes. As you work through the manual refer back to this section for help whenever you get stuck. These are only a few principles.

There are many, many more.

Chapter 4. Physical and Mental Aspects of Diabetes

Expert Care

My father took one shot of pork insulin daily, never pricked his finger to test his glucose level, and had kidney disease that went undiagnosed for several years before he succumbed to heart failure at an early age. He saw a doctor (who didn't really advise him) once every four years because that was the requirement to keep his driving privilege. My father was my first role model, and unlike him, I quickly learned I needed others. In fact, when I went to see his doctor I quickly learned I needed a different doctor.

If you don't like the care you are getting today find different caregivers. I had a diabetes doctor for years who also has Type 1. I went to him because I felt he understood how it felt to have it, which was important to me. I have had doctors with whom I did not feel any connection. One doctor asked me if I ever woke up with a low in the middle of the night, which I had (who hasn't?). After my visit, and after the driver license office put a 40 MPH restriction on my license I called his office. He said that since I had answered yes, I had had lows in the middle of the night, it meant I had lost consciousness and he naturally answered yes to the question of whether I had lost consciousness in the past few months. It felt like a set up. I didn't pass out, I woke up! It felt like I was being punished for having diabetes and I quickly searched for a doctor who would listen to me.

Another doctor spent my fifteen minutes looking at a computer screen, not talking to me. Another of my doctors didn't seem in the least interested that I made a huge transformation that helped me lower my HA1cs to the sixes and gave me my life back. I was so excited to tell him and it didn't matter a bit to him. I spoke of writing a book about my experience with diabetes. All I got was a smile.

One doctor had me go to the dietitian after we had talked for a half hour about my transformation, this book, and what I can do for others with diabetes. I told her I respected her advice but it seemed redundant to see the dietitian. I made the appointment anyway because I wanted to meet her. The dietitian wanted to know why I was even there.

"Frankly, I don't know," I said. "My doctor wanted me to see you even though I have all the information already. I teach it." We talked for an hour and made arrangements for me to come teach at her diabetes support group. She said she could not charge me for the visit because she didn't really do anything for me – instead I had done something for her.

Take control of your health care. Your doctor's duty is to help you monitor your control, order tests, and try to make sure you are following his or her instructions. When a doctor tries to treat someone who isn't in good diabetes control there is not much he can do. You are the one in charge of your care. You are the one who can change the future by taking charge of diabetes. Not your doctor.

You need to take medical matters into your own hands. Doctors, diabetes educators, dietitians, and nurse practitioners don't have time to get more involved with your care. The responsibility is on you. The primary reason people don't get the help they need from medical practitioners is that they don't want it. If you want great care, look for it and you will find it.

You have to want it

Your most conscientious, most knowledgeable, and most capable caregiver is you. You alone know when you're feeling bad, when you're being lazy about taking care of your disease, and when you need to test. You even subconsciously know what your blood sugar level is at all times.

If you take insulin, do you ever have to guess about the dosage? Guess what? You subconsciously know *what the dose needs to be*. Only your conscious mind is in the dark. If you have Type 2, and even if you do not take insulin, do you ever have to guess about your dietary intake? Guess what? Your subconscious knows that as well. Not all of us are healers by nature, but we are all capable of healing ourselves. You are your own shaman. If you don't know that or don't know how to be your own shaman, start by getting acquainted with your *inner healer*.

I have learned that I can accurately guess the correct dosage of insulin to take. How do I do it? I changed my belief from *I don't know the correct dose* to *I know the correct dose*. Now when I test and need to dose without knowing the carbohydrate count I slow down and listen. And when I listen and trust, I'm right every time. The times when I'm not correct I can always look back and see that I had not followed my own advice about the dose; my conscious thinking is louder and sometimes overrides my more intelligent, inspired subconscious, which is very quiet. I still make a few mistakes, but I recognize it and steer myself back on track.

It may seem eerie, but your body's cells actually vibrate positively or negatively in response to the knowledge in your subconscious. In fact they have more information than your conscious mind! We could write an entire book on this principle and it is somewhat difficult to grasp for the first time. For now just understand that your conscious mind is small compared to the vast knowledge of your subconscious, and it is governed by your ego.

It is your subconscious mind that governs your cells. In addition, your conscious mind is often at odds with your high-self. It's my high-self (which inhabits the subconscious) that tells me the exact insulin dose to take and my conscious *pea brain* that doubts it and occasionally wins. It wins unless I consciously choose to listen to my quieter voice – my inner healer. See the information on PSYCH-K® in Chapter 8 and the book *The Biology of Belief* by Dr. Bruce Lipton, listed in recommended reading, for more about this startling research.

Self-care is the very foundation of this volume and we have more to say throughout the book. Understand, though, that you can easily sabotage your own caregiver within, and you can also let other people sabotage you.

Healthy boundaries

For some of us the problem isn't having diabetes as much as it is dealing with the people in our lives who have an effect on us. So often we let other people encourage us to suffer and to stop pursuing what we know we want because they don't believe in our ability. Some, I'll call them dream-stealers, don't believe in achieving dreams in general.

They will usually say they just don't want to see you get hurt but at least among the ones I know that's an excuse. This is as much the case with diabetes management as it is the case with any dream, large or small. Please believe me when I say if this is what the people in your life are doing, what they say only affects you because you allow it to.

Having healthy boundaries is like having a door into your mind that you control. If you don't want to let a thought in, decide to keep it out. You may not know how to not hear it but you don't have to accept it. You don't have to *agree*. Agree to respectfully disagree. If what other people say affects you, you may have a boundary issue. Healthy personal boundaries make what others say belong to them, not you.

It's a myth that anyone can make another person feel anything. When you think another person has made you feel a certain way, check your premises. I think what really happened was that you agreed with what they said because *it's what you already say to yourself*. It's difficult enough to accept and take responsibility for diabetes. Make sure you don't allow the people in your life who have difficulty accepting your disease to cause you the same difficulty.

Where there is no door there is no way to close off outside influences. Children, for example, are easily influenced, which is like having no door to their minds. As we mature we learn to toughen our minds, which, in this analogy, is the same as installing a door. Sometimes the door swings both ways. That's how it feels when you have not established personal boundaries. Thoughts go in without being challenged.

To build boundaries when you don't have them, imagine a doorway into your mind from outside. If you imagine a latch on the door the latch will allow you to decide whether you want to let someone's comment in, in other words, to agree to let their comment be part of your beliefs. When you become able to mentally keep their opinions from being your opinions (if you don't want them to be) then you are able to filter their beliefs out. When you are unable to keep others' comments out then you are in a habit of not filtering others' beliefs, which is how they become your beliefs.

Remember, you can't believe it unless you agree to it. Instead, change the way you hear it so that others can speak their thoughts and you are able to choose to respectfully disagree. That's thought control.

One more thing: accept *you* as *you* are, whether you are sixty years old, weigh 250 lbs., have a big nose, have zits, or have a major illness like diabetes. If you find you really don't like your body use affirmations that reverse the negative thoughts about yourself. Figure out how to appreciate the attributes you don't like by asking things like, *What is the purpose of my* (fat) *legs? What is my* (big) *nose good for? What good is this* (old) *brain?* (Hint: it's much wiser than young brains). Send appreciation to the body part you have tended to put down or ignore.

Diet, Exercise, and Sleep

Sugars and simple carbohydrates cause spikes in blood sugar which we know causes a short burst of energy followed by a slump. Complex carbohydrates allow for a more even disbursement of glucose, but recent science is disputing whether even complex carbs are better. That's because complex carbs elevate the blood sugar for longer periods. Besides potentially raising your HA1c levels you could also be contributing to issues such as insulin resistance. Current research discounts the need for carbohydrates at all.

These studies point out the ineffectiveness of carbohydrates as nutritional food and endorses seriously reducing carbs altogether, whether you have diabetes or not (Gedgaudas 2011). Yes, carbs are easier on the kidneys but they contribute greatly to a myriad of the kinds of diseases that have become much more prevalent in our modern age.

pH Balance

I'm no diet expert but once I decided I wanted to learn I found some great information that helps my glucose control, which helps keep my energy high. If you have ever maintained a swimming pool you know how important pH balance is; you need to control the acid to inhibit the growth of algae, but too much alkalinity poisons the water. That's why they call it pH *balance.*

This is the balance of acidity and alkalinity in the body, which is neutral at 7.2 but experts recommend keeping it slightly more alkaline; they say you will have more energy when your pH is slightly more alkaline (but not too alkaline).

Among other forms of balance, your body works to maintain temperature, blood oxygen, and blood sugar. Your body is also in a constant state of flux between acidic and alkaline chemistry. PH balance is critical for all other systems to function normally in the body. Viruses and bacteria cannot survive in an alkaline environment but they thrive in an acidic one. On the pH scale 7 is neutral. Every number higher than 7 is 100 times more alkaline. So broccoli, with a pH of 8, is 100 times more alkaline than pure water, which is 7. Soda, at 2.5 is about 10,000 times more acidic than the body needs.

You can begin to increase alkalinity by increasing your alkaline food and water intake. That said, the digestive system is an acid system by nature. Proteins like meats undergo a change during digestion, making it OK to eat them in limited quantities without lowering pH levels greatly, even though they are high acid foods.

Potatoes, squash, brown rice and cruciferous vegetables are alkaline foods. Avocados, one of my favorite foods, are alkaline too. You can replace the water you drink, which is likely acidic, with alkaline water. You can take supplements that balance your pH. You can have your pH tested, similar to testing the pH of swimming pools. Alkaline food and water do affect your pH but so do other factors. You will find a basic pH chart for foods in Appendix A at the back of the book.

Optimal human blood pH should be maintained at slightly alkaline, between 7.35 and 7.45 according to experts. Above or below this range will be accompanied by symptoms. Acidic pH decreases the body's ability to utilize nutrients and minerals, repair cells, and detoxify heavy metals, which is why disease can take hold more easily. And bacteria and viruses thrive in an acidic environment.

Your body does a good job of regulating pH and diet is not the only determining factor in pH balance. Stress levels, toxicity levels, immune dysfunction, and oxygen/nutrient depravation can also affect pH (Alkaline Sisters).

Obesity

The relationship of diabetes to obesity may not be as we tend to think. Obesity itself may not be as much of a diabetes risk factor as we thought. It may be genetic in nature and a symptom of insulin resistance, rather than its cause. Or they both may be symptoms of our modern diet that is too heavily dependent on carbohydrates. See Appendix B for more information on this subject.

Regardless of the cause of Type 2 diabetes, it cannot be shown that obesity causes diabetes. And the belief that obesity causes diabetes contributes to the notion that while the public may feel somewhat sympathetic to people with Type 2 there is an underlying feeling that they brought it on themselves.

No one deserves to have diabetes so don't judge yourself by the same harsh standards society does. While there are stories about people who lost the weight and their diabetes disappeared, the ideas we discuss in further chapters, things like straightening out the DIS-ease in your life, losing weight, changing your diet, and getting the education needed to reverse diabetes, can help you become happy, healthy, and in control, without all the added drama lots of people with diabetes go through.

Exercise

It's time to look at your own physical energy to begin to solve your energy problems. If you find you eat the wrong foods it often means your will-power is low, you just don't feel like doing much, and energy-wise you are taking big gulps. Believe it or not, choosing to remain in your comfort zone can exhaust your energy. Over-doing rest feeds tiredness. You can be out of balance by working too hard and not resting and you can be out of balance by only resting and not working.

The answer is exercise. Since cardio-vascular exercise increases heart, lung, and blood hemoglobin capacity, and strength exercise increases muscle capacity, both types of exercise actually increase energy. The increase is obvious with routine exercise over time.

Like the folks at Nike say, *Just do it!* You will increase your confidence, feel energized, tighten your control, and have more spring in your step. And you will live longer.

Rest

Think about the amount of physical and mental energy you use. If you run a mile you know your energy is zapped and you need to rest. Working mentally for four hours straight at the computer has the effect of zapping your energy too; it's just that your energy is low in a different way – mentally. Mental energy depletes quickly and unwittingly.

You probably don't need to remember to take a ten minute break after running a few miles, but you will have to consciously remember to take a ten-minute break every 90-120 minutes at your workplace, wherever it happens to be. Do what you can to restore your mental energy balance.

Sleep

When centenarians, people who have reached age 100, are asked "What is the secret to long life?" the first thing they say is "Not dying." But the next thing they usually say is *sleep*. The older we get the more sleep we need, but research also points to sleep as the one thing you can do now to add years to your life.

Sleep deprivation shortens lives but it also steals energy. And you know low energy fosters bad behaviors; depending on your personality when your energy is low you may become lazy at testing or prone to angry outbursts. You may eat to self-medicate or go into depression because of it. People with sleep disorders need to take a close look at the underlying cause. Difficulty sleeping is almost always a symptom of some DIS-ease.

What to do about low energy

Mentally, you cannot renew your energy and using it in an unbalanced way is like taking *big gulps* of energy. Preserve it with periodic breaks of at least 10 minutes every two hours. During the break do the opposite of what you were doing; if you were sitting, stand and walk. If you were focused on a computer screen, focus on the horizon. If you were inside go outside. And drink lots of water (not soda or energy drinks). You will notice an increase in energy.

People often say, "I'm just a mess." But that statement is too general to do you any good. By pinpointing the source of your low energy you can get to the real problem. If you have low energy it will help to look at your patterns. Is it seasonal? You may need to address patterns that occur at specific times of the year. To keep your energy from decreasing even more, regardless of the cause of it, do something completely different from what you are doing.

Where I live we have cold, inverted winters and by February I used to get extreme cabin fever. To help fight depression I began working in my garden as soon as the ground begins to thaw; in the garden I can watch flowers beginning to become alive again. What could you do that's opposite? If you tend to crawl into your cave, go out. Don't want to talk? Call someone. Don't want to feel the cold? Go for a walk in the wind.

If you feel guilty resting, let curling up and watching an old movie be your reward for hard work, and don't allow guilt to stop you – it's your reward. You can increase your energy by rewarding yourself. Allowing rewards can create a wonderful transformation. I used to pay my kids to not burn down the house while I was away. Some said it was inappropriate and for a while I allowed that to stop me. But giving kids rewards for staying safe felt good and I changed my paradigm and became a person who gives myself and others rewards for everyday accomplishments. It's a great way to restore energy.

Your body tells you when you are out of balance so structure your program with built-in balance. When you are confident in your decisions no matter what people say, you begin to know who you are and where you are going, which rewards you with the highest energy of all. The better you understand that you are already enough the better you will be at giving without the need to receive anything in return. You will also begin to receive without feeling you need to reciprocate. And all that synergy creates energy.

Taking charge of your emotions, changing your beliefs, and getting your spirituality on track will make everything else so easy that you'll actually do it. As you develop your personal system, keep in mind all of the ways you can increase, restore, and preserve your energy. This will lead you to a place in your life where taking care of diabetes feels like it's not work at all.

Becoming a vibrant and energetic person who happens to have diabetes will require increased energy; you will begin to have more energy as you become more vibrant. It's an upward spiraling cycle. So establish a plan for accomplishing that goal. My map will help but you will need to incorporate many things, most importantly, a big WHY. Once you have your WHY it's only a matter of following a few proven principles. You, in turn, will be able to achieve any goal, whether the goal is becoming happy with diabetes or healing diabetes altogether.

Chapter 5. The Emotional Rollercoaster

There is nothing either good or bad but thinking makes it so.
~William Shakespeare

Before we can become different we have to change the way we think about what it is we want to change, and the way you think about it is reflected in the way you feel about it. I spend a lot of time on emotions because it's where people have the most trouble. It's your emotional state that lets diabetes rule you.

We've discussed emotions in terms of the musical scale. Now let's dive deeper to see why emotions have such a profound effect on people they literally stop us from living... they stop us from taking action. Ultimately we lose out on better health. We'll begin with some of the ways diabetes toys with our emotions. Just being aware can make the difference between overpowering diabetes and being overpowered by it.

Ask yourself, "How am I spending emotional energy?" Some people live their entire lives in an emotionally exhausted condition, rarely more so than with diabetes. The more you allow yourself to feel defeated the more energy you will spend. Giving conscious and unconscious attention to worry and anxiety zaps energy. Instead, focus as best you can on the positive things in your life. You will immediately feel more vitality. The more time you spend in peace, harmony, and love the more energy you will have by default; you'll preserve energy because you will not be using so much of it.

Minefields

High glucose levels, both slight and excessive, affect anxiety. And lows affect it too. Highs or lows can feel uncomfortable; high blood-sugar can cause mood changes while low blood sugar can affect your ability to concentrate, which can make you feel grouchy. So glucose levels can affect emotions and emotions also can affect glucose levels and diabetes control. It's a nasty cycle.

Blood sugar spikes when your body releases stress hormones. The stress of public speaking, tight work deadlines, or bungee jumping causes blood-sugar to significantly increase, even in people without diabetes. This is because in the body's normal fight-or-flight response the liver releases glucose to make energy available to the cells.

People with diabetes either do not have insulin available to let the glucose into their cells when it spikes like this, or they have cells that are resistant to the insulin. So when we are under stress, sugar builds up in the blood. The same effect occurs when we are sick with a fever or the flu, and sometimes when our blood sugar drops to low levels.

Blame keeps people from taking responsibility for their future. But prejudice is another kind of blame that makes life even harder for many with Type 2. Most are overweight and live inactive lifestyles. Many researchers believe that obesity is probably not the cause of Type 2 – it's more of a symptom. But society blames people with Type 2 Diabetes for not living more active lifestyles – being *lazy* – because they think exercise and losing weight could have prevented it.

It's natural to have a bad day, feel angry, or resent "healthy" people. Those feelings come with the package. But if you are angry and short-tempered, or if you're depressed all of the time, you will have a much harder time taking good care of yourself. If you have a serious problem with any of the emotions that come with diabetes, get help. This goes for partners of people with diabetes, and for parents of children with diabetes as well.

Stressors

The stresses in your life that contributed to the onset of diabetes are probably the same ones that inhibit good control and a positive attitude toward your life now. However, new stressors often show up that hinder further success. I have identified the major ones that limit good diabetes control, and specifically the ones that limited my control on Page 8. We will drill down beneath each one in these chapters. The list is by no means comprehensive, but it will serve to help you begin to see the role stress plays in not taking good care of yourself.

For now just identify your stressors as best you can. See whether some of them are obvious. Take out a pen and write down something that stresses you, whether physically, mentally, emotionally, or socially; describe what it does and the effect it has on your control. Then see if you can identify more. Go!

_____

_____

_____

_____

_____

_____

_____

_____

_____

_____

_____

There are many pressures we do battle with every day. Let's talk about a few of them. Throughout the remainder of the book you will receive guidance on how to address them.

Anger: Anger keeps you from moving forward, especially when every time you try to think positively about your control you feel angry. The feeling keeps you stuck wishing you didn't have diabetes and unable to do what needs to be done. Anger about other things can affect diabetes control too.

Anxiety: Anxiety causes you to become overwhelmed and to shut down, keeping you from being proactive about diabetes. Anxiety about diabetes creates a negative perspective, which in turn, often creates negative actions.

Resentment: Resentment keeps you from feeling confident. Who can feel confident with a 100 pound ball chained to them? Resentment makes positive steps seem impossible.

Worry: As with anxiety, worry keeps you from being proactive. Worrying about it may make you better at diet, testing, and exercise, but it won't help you like your life any better. Worry may make you cynical and stubborn.

Apathy: Obviously, apathy keeps you from acting to take care of yourself. Over time apathy is the biggest killer of people with diabetes. As everyone knows, the greater the apathy about a disease the lower the ability to manage it.

Pain/bad day: Both of these problems lead to doing things to comfort yourself. People do not indulge nearly as much when they are having a good day and are not in pain. When we are in pain we often self-medicate with drugs, alcohol, or other things. Eating to feel better is as bad for people with diabetes as drugs and alcohol are for everybody.

Guilt: Guilt may make you self-medicate to feel better. The low energy produced by guilt causes you to be more prone to temptation creating a downward spiral of poor control aggravated by the guilt.

Shock: Being in shock about some event causes your physiological functions to shut down. The shock of diagnosis causes some people to lose perspective on life and to give up. Other types of shock, like divorce or the death of a loved one, can cause similar effects.

Resistance: Resisting anything keeps you in a defensive posture. In fight mode you can see only a few options. The opposite of fighting is to surrender. Surrendering to the fact of diabetes means you stop fighting it. Then you can become open to new possibilities for your happiness.

Too tired: Like apathy, tiredness keeps you from acting to take care of yourself. Thoughts like "I'll test it later," "I just want to lay here for a while," or "I'll eat this just once" easily creep in when you are tired.

Victim: Being a victim causes you to not take responsibility for managing your disease and stops your ability to control your own disease due to an unwillingness to own it. If it's someone else fault why should you have to take care of it? Even if you think you're not doing this check again. It's subtle. When do you know you have stopped being a victim? When you feel you have power over whatever it is that victimized you, which in this case is diabetes.

Grief: As with anger, grief keeps you from moving forward in life because you are still mourning your lost health. Being stuck in grief keeps you from taking action to change your circumstances. Later I will devote an entire section on the subject of grief.

Doubt: Failure stops people from making progress. Fear and doubt caused by limiting beliefs about your ability and your own resourcefulness can keep you from asking better questions, seeking proactive solutions, and being persistent.

Vulnerability/Embarrassment/Isolation/Shame: The first three of these cause fear and contribute to the hiding behaviors that result from the shame. Your first response is to try to hide whatever it is you think people see that makes you feel vulnerable. You isolate yourself, then you feel alone, then you self-medicate (which makes you feel worse), then you feel guilty, which often causes you to isolate yourself more.

Cravings: Cravings result from unmet needs. Whether dietary or emotional, unmet needs trigger the hunger centers of your brain. For me, cravings begin when I feel deprived and unable to do something everyone else can. People often become obsessed about one thing to the exclusion of everything else. When you give in to it the three-year-old (your ego) is in charge.

Compulsiveness: Cravings often become compulsive when you are out of touch with yourself and feeling too tired to resist. When the three-year-old is in charge and you don't have enough energy to stop it, control becomes nearly impossible. That's the definition of a compulsion.

Attitude: That feeling that you are fine, that you have completed your work on diabetes control, and that you have arrived at some conclusive result may be stopping you from fully living. When you think you're fine you don't continue to work at improving whatever it is that could be even better.

Stubbornness: Stubbornness keeps you closed to new solutions. This is often the result of not thinking you need outside help. Un-teachable people desire to remain closed to new solutions and ideas. They believe they know as much as anyone else. They are unwilling to take new steps toward a more positive change. This is an excuse.

Poor will-power: A common symptom of diabetes is low energy, and frustration about it lowers energy even more. When your energy is low so is your will-power. You cannot force yourself to have more will power either. Increase your energy and you will automatically have more power over your cravings, compulsions, and attitudes. There are many ways to begin to increase your energy.

Common emotional baggage

Emotional baggage consists of feelings that have become so normal-feeling that you don't notice them anymore. They are the ratty old coat you may be wearing even though it's smelly and full of holes, because you have always worn it and that makes it comfortable. Here I list examples of common emotional baggage.

Negative self talk and low confidence. Everyone who has negative self-talk has low confidence but it's often hard to recognize; we tend to have a high tolerance for it. Most people don't know they can minimize and even eliminate negative self-talk; they don't know what it would feel like to be rid of it. I use to believe this inner negativity was part of being human.

Negative self-talk is like Tinnitus – ringing in your ears. If you have it you are not aware of it all the time, but when you think about it you hear it. I have never been able to eliminate Tinnitus but I learned to live in harmony with it. Negative self-talk is a lot like Tinnitus, but unlike Tinnitus, there *is* something you can do about it. You don't have to live with it. Why?

Because negative-self talk is merely a bad habit.

Why are people in marriages and jobs they hate? Why do people feel unloved? Why is there so much poverty in the world? Disapproving self-talk is the plague of the earth – it's an epidemic. It's like an audio tape loop that plays over and over in your head feeding you dark thoughts about yourself, other people, and your world. At least eighty per cent of the people I mentor are stuck because of low confidence and negative thoughts. I had them; I still hear them from time to time trying to undermine my confidence, but I have beaten them into submission. I am the one in charge, not the voices in my head.

Self-criticism keeps confidence low. On the outside it looks harmless enough, you are trying to toughen yourself up by criticizing yourself, believing it's a form of self-preservation. But it's really a double-edged sword. When you are in the negative feedback loop you are completely un-nurturing, unloving, and uncaring to yourself, ways of thinking which can never make you tough.

Confidence Curve

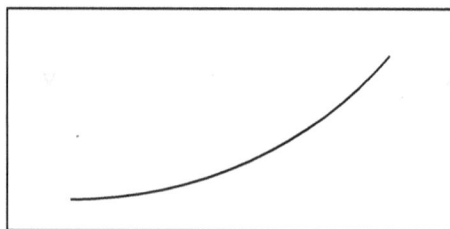

Starts slow   Builds   Builds faster

Just like a learning curve, the confidence curve is gradual; but you can become more confident each day. Begin by creating new self-talk as we have discussed. After a week you'll feel better... after a month even better... and only a few months later confidence has fully become a habit. Confidence may start slow, but with time it builds, increasing in speed and decreasing in difficulty.

Emotional exhaustion. Thinking negatively about yourself uses a lot of energy. In Chapter 3 we discussed four sources of energy. You have a fixed amount of energy for physical, emotional, mental, and spiritual activities. You can easily see ways you exhaust physical energy. You can replenish physical and mental exhaustion with diet, exercise, and rest. Mentally you become exhausted when you work at mental tasks too hard without taking breaks.

Emotional exhaustion can be chronic if you have a lot of self-recrimination, you live in fear, or you feel angry much of the time; the worse you feel the more it drains you. It's a downward spiral because when you're tired your thoughts automatically go negative, using up what little energy you have. Positive emotions use little energy by comparison. The first step is to recognize your emotional exhaustion. Next, understand that you can choose a better way. You don't have to live your life exhausted.

Sensitivity. Some of us are more feeler than thinker. It's a certain personality trait of at least half the population. If you are a feeler-type (motivated by love, as discussed earlier), discouraging words will set you off emotionally. You want to let someone else's words roll off your back but you can't. Everything goes in; the things they say and even the things you think they might be thinking, and there is no pre-installed mental filter to stop it.

Fortunately, in this case, you can install a filter yourself. You can be a powerful feeler-healer by working through low confidence that keeps you stuck. Stop being hurt every time other people push your buttons. You will still be a feeler with the challenges this level of sensitivity brings, but you don't have to be derailed by it every time.

Everyone can develop mental toughness. As we discussed, start by imagining a latch on the door of your mind. Now, rather than immediately reacting, you want to stop and think about it, which is a responsive action. "Do I agree or not? It doesn't match my new image of myself. That's you, not me." That's being mentally tough.

Frustration. If you get frustrated a lot you allow things to bother you. Frustration comes from telling yourself something is unacceptable. Usually you want something to happen faster or things aren't going as well as you wish they would. In reality, there's some element you are resisting.

Because becoming frustrated is a habit it takes work to change it. Literally, to form a new habit requires a new neural pathway. When you feel overwhelmed it's like your mind flips to an old, worn path. You have to be persistent; creating a new pathway takes a conscious effort of new thinking repeatedly.

You will eventually form a new habit of thinking. To do this when you feel overwhelmed you can say, "I have had confidence and I can have it again." The new path becomes the one you use by habit once you become successful at not going back to your old thinking.

Impatience. If you find you are often impatient, take another look at what you are trying to accomplish. If you hate something it will frustrate you every time, so figure out how not to hate it. Figure out what's good about it. I did this with diabetes and before that I did it with my household finances. Also, focus on every small success, and if it helps you, write about your individual successes. When you feel frustrated go back and read them. If you look back over time—from the first time you began a particular project – you can see what's changed.

Confusion. Whenever you are confused there is something you are not willing to admit or face. I have helped many people face what they fear and get over the confusion. If you are confused about any part of your illness it will keep you stuck. But confusion is helpful if you recognize it; now, when I feel confused, I make myself look at the situation as objectively as I can to understand what it is I am avoiding looking at or pretending not to see.

Control. It's interesting that whenever I encounter someone who is *controlling* I can see that they don't feel as though they have control, but they don't know it. They seem to me to be pretending not to see it. If you find yourself wanting to control situations and people, the problem is with you. Take out a blank sheet of paper and draw a fairly large circle – four or five inches in diameter. Inside the circle name everything over which you have real control. Place everything over which you have no control outside the circle. Name everything you can think of; finances, health, your partner, your actions, anger, your children, the weather, your thoughts, your body, diabetes, God, pizza. Fill up the page with things both inside and outside the circle.

Inside the circle you should have written only the things contained within you – your thoughts, your creations, your actions, buying pizza, eating pizza, and your perceptions, prayers, gratitude, character, and so on. Outside the circle would be all the rest; nature, God, other people, events, other creations, the pizza. How well did you do at knowing what you really do and do not control?

Trying to control people is frustrating because you cannot control them, just as they can't control you – unless you let them. The same goes for events like an accident caused by someone or something else. But you do have control over how you perceive it, feel about it, decide, think, and feel about it, and the actions you take in response to it. That's the only control you can possibly have. Attempts to control anything outside the circle will be frustrating. This principle is the key to learning how to stop feeling like a powerless victim and start feeling powerful.

Understand what triggers your need to control. What is the underlying need? You probably feel you have no control so you need a sense of control. Instead, what if you do not need to have control? Would that help overcome the problem of not having control?

Let's look at a situation with another person. You may have felt forced into something over which you had no say, and it made you angry. What if you gave in and did the thing? *But then the other person would win.* What would be terrible about that? Would the world fly apart? You'd feel insecure; you'd feel vulnerable. Nobody wants to be a victim but plenty of people whom we view as victims don't feel at all that they are victims. Your level of victimhood depends on your mental, emotional, spiritual, and physical responses to people and situations.

Other people do not do things the same as you do no matter how much you want them to. It might not be right according to you, but you have zero control over that. You can influence them to a point, and you can understand it, but you can't make them do what you would do or make them change their thoughts, feelings, and behaviors. It may take effort but it could bring profound change if you were to start to risk, in small ways, not having control. What can you do with the contrary, frustrated feelings? Release them. We'll show you how in Chapter 8.

Past thinking. If you find your thoughts often go back to the past you can expect to be constantly frustrated. This is *now* and the *past* is over. If you can move into thinking about the present, and even the future, you will have much different outcomes.

Deserving. Many of us have been taught "it's better to give than to receive," and I believe it's true. But we have learned from that thought or something similar, that it's selfish to want what we desire. Airline flight attendants teach setting your own oxygen mask in place before helping your loved ones. The Bible says first *fill up your own cup.* If you aren't fulfilled yourself you limit what you are able to give.

Next, let go of your guilt; guilt doesn't serve others any more than it serves you. Before I learned to *deserve* the things I want I was trying to give and I mostly felt exhausted from the effort and guilty about not doing as much as I wanted to do. Since my own needs weren't met I was actually more selfish, which brought on more guilt.

Who's going to meet your needs? *You are.* Imagine if you were filled to overflowing; you would automatically want to give. That's giving from your abundance. Change your belief to one that really serves your higher purposes. Do things for yourself and you will naturally do more for others too.

Overwhelmed by feelings. Overwhelming feelings trigger emotional responses like crying and fits of anger. What are you doing to take care of yourself at those times? Some people feel a constant bombardment of feelings, making it hard to stay on track and do the work of becoming healthy. First, ask yourself, *how high is my expectation of where I should be?* Is it too high? Does this thing I expect need to happen all at once? There will come a time when all of this work will begin to click. So if you are overwhelmed about anything, slow down, breathe, and relax. You'll feel better and be better able to focus.

Emotional eating. Many people with or without diabetes fall into emotional eating when their energy becomes too low, and people fall into a chronic habit of emotional eating when low energy is chronic. For many, emotional eating becomes a vicious cycle that they don't know how to stop.

Will-power doesn't work; you need to get at the problem below the surface of emotional eating. I had an eating disorder that never existed until after I was diagnosed. For me, anger and resentment took my energy straight to the bottom; I felt crummy about myself, then I self-medicated with junk food because I hated to do anything I felt forced into doing. I knew I had a problem, I didn't want to talk about it, and I could not solve it without help. If emotional eating is a problem for you there are books, programs, instructors, counsellors and coaches who are ready to help. Get help.

Perfectionism. Perfectionism plagues a large cross section of society; it results from low confidence and inner voices telling you incessantly that you aren't good enough. No matter how well you do you can never win the perfectionism game. *You can never win*; and *never* is a word I try *never* to use.

Perfectionism at its core is based in frustration and fear. Remember, for change to occur you must move to a different level; the level above perfection is excellence. Excellence is higher than perfection because perfection is an illusion. We're human, which, by definition, means we're not perfect and never can be. So needing yourself, someone else, or anything to be perfect can only result in heartache.

Perfectionists waiver back and forth between perfectionism and excellence. When you feel a sense of accomplishment you have moved to excellence. Don't undo it by discounting the feeling. Excellence gives you peace and acceptance. Acceptance is the highest emotion. When you feel anxious, ask "How can I feel peace and acceptance?" "What can I find that's good about this situation?" The only perfect thing you can have is excellence.

You might feel like you aren't improving quickly enough. A voice in your head may say, "You have to do better!" Realize it's a DIS-ease you will *never* overcome as long as you give in to it.

If perfectionism governs you, begin to recover by letting things be a little *imperfect*. Keep doing what you are doing even if you are frustrated. Pat yourself on the back for even your small achievements. Be proud that you are keeping at it when it gets difficult. If you need more help with perfectionism see our list of resources in the back of the book. You will find a great book entitled *Too Perfect: When Being in Control Gets Out of Control* (Mallinger and DeWyze, 1992).

Sadness. Not only does diabetes increase the risk of serious health complications, but uncontrolled diabetes also may worsen depression, another vicious cycle. Depression is a necessary process that can go on too long. The most effective tool for sadness and depression is action. Do something. Move.

Many people do not have clinical depression but they become depressed from time to time. Learn to recognize the signs early. It may feel like a ping pong game in your head that keeps you awake at night. The best remedy is changing your focus from what you don't have to what you have. If that doesn't work, get up, drink a glass of water or a brew a cup of tea, and start writing about what's bothering you. Let the little cloud park over your head for a little while. Love this valid part of you. But don't let the cloud stay for good. Don't dwell on thinking that your work isn't working.

Depression is always accompanied by low self-confidence. It is both a cause and an effect. It may make you self-medicate to comfort yourself. Try using affirmations that deal with exactly what you tell yourself to begin to turn depression around (see Chapter 8 for help creating affirmations). If you can't get a handle on depression, please seek professional help. And remember, you can do it.

Dependence, Independence, and Interdependence

Codependency. Codependency is a form of dysfunctional dependence. You didn't have to come from an alcoholic family to have a life characterized by codependency. Some conditions of dysfunctional families continue to painfully influence peoples' self-feelings, attitudes, and behaviors throughout their lives. Codependent people are adult children; in a codependent family parental roles are reversed in such a way that the parent acts like a child and the child takes on the role of parent. Someone has to be the parent, right?

If you learn you are from a family characterized by these role reversals your dysfunctional relationships will finally begin to make sense. You will find that the mental defenses you use, defenses you built to protect yourself when you were a child, were the result of a child's inability to change the physical circumstances of his or her family.

"I never knew how my dad was going to be. I had to walk on egg-shells. Now it's causing issues," is typical of someone raised in this type of dysfunctional family. You do not have to remain a victim. From childhood you learned a habit. Now it's time to unlearn it; it no longer serves you, and worse, it's hurting you.

Forgive yourself for thoughts, beliefs, and behaviors that you no longer subscribe to. Research books and programs on codependency to get help in turning your relationships and your life back around. Choose the direction you want to be facing.

Interdependence. Normally we move from dependence to independence. First, we are dependent children, the natural immature state, and then we move to independence, which is our natural mature state. Dr. Steven R. Covey refers to a third ultimate state of interdependence that some people move into, which is characterized by giving back and becoming connected with the world. Here you become an excellent giver *and* receiver. Not everyone achieves interdependence but everyone can. It's important when building your ideal system because spiritual well-being thrives in the connected environment of interdependency.

Emotional Growth

What can you do about dark emotions? When you're angry, depressed, moody, sad, and down on yourself it's hard to stop feeling that way. When you feel low it zaps your energy and brings out your worst; you worry, beat yourself up, criticize others, hate your circumstances, and more. I hate to be the one to say it, and there is really only one way to say this; chronic dark emotions come from a low, stuck place from which you emit words, feelings, and actions.

Most people grow up physically without even thinking much about it; we go through the stages of childhood, adolescence, and adulthood dealing with the challenges each stage brings. But emotional growth can be stunted by ourselves or brought on by circumstances in our lives; circumstances that are usually traumatic. Emotional growth means taking responsibility for your feelings. You take responsibility not by blame but by acknowledgment. This must be undertaken by you and no one else. To explain this we'll go back to the anger that kept me stuck for over twenty years. I desperately needed to work through my anger but it was too scary and I didn't want to.

The result of not wanting to do the hard part was that it made my life more difficult until I did. But once I went through the pain of treating it, feeling my emotions rather than suppressing them, I was able to mature emotionally. For me that meant that in my thirties when I was ready to, I began to experience emotionally all the stages of adolescence and young adult maturity, starting with when I was around age ten and ending when I reached an emotional age that matched my physical age. It wasn't easy but I could not be whole until I did it.

I could not see my own immaturity, though others saw it. For most people emotional maturity comes naturally. But some of us become stuck and must make a conscious effort to grow up emotionally. It can be a very scary process, and rough. For most people who are emotionally immature it's too scary and they feel they have no choice but to remain stuck – or don't even realize that they are actually stuck. It's usually not a conscious choice; we had no idea we were choosing immaturity over maturity.

Those who have this issue and who don't do the work necessary to grow up emotionally have low energy with no inclination to change. It takes a lot of energy to mature emotionally and they don't have very much energy. If you want to choose a better life, get professional counseling. Remember to love and nurture yourself and to surround yourself with supportive people to hold you accountable *and* to hold your hand.

I will not try to name every tendency that gets in peoples' way but if you see some tendencies you have that you may have forgotten, add them to your list. Remember the list that began this chapter. Fill it in if the topics here have triggered anything for you. If discovering your tendencies is new territory for you, join the club.

This work is all about your commitment to yourself and your trust and confidence in your ability to be the director of your life. You are learning what you need to know and to do in order to become free from suffering with diabetes. And what you need to know and do to become free from suffering with diabetes is also what you need to live a full, wholesome life.

If you know a certain tendency that's stopping you, you can recognize it, stop doing it, and decide not to do it anymore. There is no right or wrong way, only tools. You will know the direction in which you want to move by what comes to mind to work on next. You will have the tools, you will know how it works, and you will be able to do it.

Chapter 6. Grief, Anger, and Fear

Three common and difficult emotions, grief, anger, and fear, seem to cause more suffering for people with diabetes than all the rest. I have not been the only one to get stuck in emotions when it came to overcoming my personal challenges. Whether it's diabetes or some other trial, many of us tend to get stuck. I hope this chapter will help you see grief, anger, and fear from a different perspective, as well as to help you see it as a natural process, which will help you move forward again.

My Wakeup call

Vulnerability is a powerful tool. Allow me to be a bit vulnerable (again) as I relate my story about finding myself at the *Bitter End* (a fitting name).

This is the story of when I woke up. I had had diabetes for a while – but I woke up to the fact that I wasn't taking care of it and I woke up to why. I realized a lot of things – not only that I hated it. I was terrified of it. And it was there that I faced my own mortality for the very first time.

This awakening occurred on a Caribbean sailboat cruise. I get seasick on boats so I went prepared, or at least I thought I had prepared.

I had seasickness patches to put behind my ear and Dramamine as a backup. The problem with the patches, though, was they were new (in fact they were later recalled because they were too strong).

I began using the patches by not following the directions. I put the patch on after we set sail, while the instructions said to put it on six hours before. Then after just a few minutes I began to feel like I was having an anxiety attack or a caffeine overdose. I felt so buzzed I couldn't stand it, so I removed the patch.

A while later I started to feel sick and then, later, I couldn't hold anything down. I had Dramamine, but once everything starts coming up it's all over with the Dramamine. I really did not have a good enough back-up plan in case the patch didn't work, so by the end of the second day I was endlessly hurling over the side of the boat. Our friends became troubled and embarrassed for me. As it turned out, they weren't great friends.

Finally in the middle of the night I was on deck trying to feel better and not having any luck. An important point here is that I had not even brought along anything to test my sugar. That was my first awakening – I was too unconcerned about diabetes. I was going on a sailboat, I knew I get sick on boats, I thought I'd be OK with the patch, I didn't think I needed my glucometer, and I didn't have a back-up plan. I had not come prepared to take care of my illness and it was perhaps the stupidest, most dangerous move I have ever made.

My husband came up on deck and found me in poor condition. He woke up the captain and said, "We need to get her off the boat and find help." We were at a place in the British Virgin Islands called the Bitter End. It was a small resort at the end of the string of islands with a restaurant, a bar, and condos. That was all.

I was a wretched retching wreck.

The captain motored us to shore and went back to the boat. We went in search of help but the entire resort was closed up tight as a drum. Not a sound and not a person in sight – anywhere. Nobody to wake up, no one to call for emergency, no one to help. Only then, when it was too late, did I realize my second big mistake: I had not even brought my insulin off the boat! And there was no way to call the captain – the boat was too far out and there were no cell phones in those days. So we stayed on the beach for the longest night of our lives, and I was sicker than I have ever been.

It hurts to think about how sick I was. I blamed myself for my stupidity – it was so naïve to have brought myself to this bitter end. My throat felt ragged. I lay on a beach chair regretting that I had not brought insulin, regretting not having even brought my meter, regretting my life, diabetes, and everything else I could possibly lament. I knew that besides being seasick my blood sugar was through the roof. In the high hundreds, I guessed. If you know diabetes you know that's the kind of blood sugar high that causes a coma. I drifted in and out of consciousness. Glade said I moaned all night and every few minutes I leaned over my chair again and, even though there was absolutely nothing left in my stomach, I retched again.

As dawn finally approached my husband tried to wave to the boat and finally about six in the morning he got their attention and the captain came to shore. Glade said, "I need you to go back to the boat and get my wife's insulin and then I need you to leave us here on shore for a while so we can bring her sugar down." That was back in the days when insulin took about two hours to start to work, not like the faster insulin we have now. I'd had diabetes for about ten years and I had no idea how to bring down a really high blood sugar quickly, or how really to treat this disease.

And I'll tell you the hardest reality I woke up to then – *I was clueless because I'd been too angry about having diabetes to learn what I needed to know.* This "non-learning" had hurt me for the ten years that I'd lived with diabetes, and it was devastating to me now. And this is what I faced that night. I was stuck in grief and finding myself helpless to save my own life.

Nobody but *me* was going fix diabetes; it was up to *me* to save my life.

If you are still in mourning about diabetes, take time now to address all your issues related to anger and grief about having it; otherwise this is what's probably going to kill you. Address it or stay stuck in grief and die.

Let's go through the various stages that people stuck in grief experience. After that I will give you tools to help you through the grieving process once and for all. And once that's done you can begin to get on with the rest of your life, but only once you do it.

Resolving Grief

If you feel you are moving forward then you may not have suppressed emotions; if you are stuck, you are suppressing. Many people resist their emotions but if you release your feelings you will again be able to move forward and get your life back on track.

If you recognize you are stuck look at diabetes grief like grieving for other losses, like the loss of a loved one. You must mourn your lost health and vitality just as you would mourn death, terminal illness, and any other tragedy.

Psychologists refer to universal stages of grieving that are our natural response to terminal illness, chronic illness, and death, whether your response is to your own or another person's event. The order of denial, anger, bargaining, depression and acceptance, is typical. However, you might move through the stages in a different order, or move in and out of stages; in other words, if you have worked through anger you could find yourself back at anger again later. Remember that people spend varying lengths of time in various stages. But if you don't feel as though you are moving through a stage you may be stuck at that stage.

1. Denial. The first reaction to a diagnosis of diabetes is typically to deny the seriousness of the situation. In my case I did not want to acknowledge that what I wanted to do about it, which was to not take it seriously, was not going to work. Denial is usually temporary and hopefully you have moved through it. In my case I worked through it, went through a pregnancy taking full responsibility, then moved back into denial afterwards. If you have not fully accepted the seriousness of diabetes you have denial.

2. Anger. People with diabetes feel angry that there is no cure; it feels unfair, nobody can fix it, and that means imprisonment for the rest of your life. The result is that many people are stuck in anger, and feel as though the only thing left to do is to suffer while they wait for a cure. They are trying to put off the inevitable while waiting for the slow and hideous death they always hear about. But you can process your anger by moving through it. Peace and diabetes *can* co-exist.

3. Bargaining. When control has been wrestled from you it leaves you feeling vulnerable. To regain control you may have tried some form of bargaining. And you may have looked at it as ownership. Taking ownership is one of the important tools I used to come to a place of authenticity with my disease. But my first attempt to take ownership was misplaced. I realized I could have sought help for depression and I could have taken better steps to manage anxiety earlier in life, before the onset of diabetes. But I had not done that. In my case I desperately wished I could go back in time and change the past; of course that type of bargaining is useless.

4. Depression. Depression occurs when our efforts to bargain, or to reconcile our anger and pain, aren't working so we give up. You may already have had depression prior to diagnosis, as I did. If so, consult a doctor, get counseling, and take anti-depressants if necessary, but sort through it. Do the work on depression by moving, connecting with people you love, and taking steps in the direction you intuitively know to take. Steps you probably don't want to take. Steps which will be outside your comfort zone.

5. Acceptance. With diabetes we tend to wander in and out of acceptance; we may feel acceptance of it one day, or even for a time, and then move back again to anger and denial. Acceptance doesn't mean the same as happiness in this sense, but acceptance takes different forms. Once you know how, you can move to a level of acceptance of diabetes where you will find peace and calmness without having to suffer – there is no suffering with acceptance in this highest form.

How to move past grief so you can move on

Once you understand grief better you can identify it by the low energy that comes with it; it will be much easier to recognize your grief and recognizing it is the key to moving through it. We talked earlier about letting go of emotions as you become aware you are holding onto them. Emotions are not long lasting; in fact, they are extremely short-lived and are gone in the very next moment.

If you find your emotions are lasting, however, check to see if it's the memory of the recent emotion you are experiencing. Is it the memory of how you felt just a moment ago? Is it a feeling that has lingered for days, weeks or even months?

There is a subtle difference between the emotion of now and the memory of an emotion you felt earlier. You will notice this difference once you become aware that in the next moment what you feel is actually from an instant memory of the feeling you just had. Dark emotions that last for months and even years are memories. They become worry, dread, depression, fear, and anxiety. With practice you can limit and even eliminate these memory emotions from your future.

Try the Sedona method on grief's denial, anger, bargaining, and depression feelings (Dwoskin, 2003) and see whether the feeling is lessened or even gone completely. If it's not gone you should notice it's at least lighter. Then go through the steps again; you may be surprised that a different emotion comes up the second time. Simply ask yourself what you are feeling this moment or what your present emotion is. You will find basic instructions in Chapter 8.

There are many methods for working through emotions. People tend to complicate things as a general rule and it's this tendency to complicate our emotions that causes us to stay stuck in them. To keep from feeling the pain of some events and thoughts we suppress them rather than expressing them. Some people find it very cathartic to write down their thoughts – to let them out by releasing them onto paper. Or you might try drawing them, writing a poem about them, or any combination of these approaches.

Moving through grief does not need to be complicated or difficult, but it's plenty difficult for many people who live with grief. It's as difficult as you make it. After making my own life messier by going about it the hard way I finally learned how easy it truly can be if I *let* it be easy. To do this the easy way, regardless of what method you use, recognize the five stages of grief as you move in and out of them. You will move through them by expressing them rather than suppressing them (which is the same as holding on to them). Going through them, not suppressing them, is the easy way.

Boiling Mad

You don't know it but...

It's hard to imagine that very many people are as obstinate as I was and the story about my trip to the bitter end of the Caribbean is most likely the exception and not the rule. However, if you recognize yourself in any part of my story please take some time to address your anger about diabetes and start to take steps to resolve it. This one factor will add many years and exceptional quality to your life.

I once worked with a woman who had diabetes for fifteen years. She was in her thirties but she looked sixty. She obviously had given up on herself and her life, since she kept large Butterfinger bars in her desk and it was all she ever seemed to eat. Once I asked her what her blood sugars were and she said she didn't know; she never tested. I asked her how much insulin she was taking and she said fifteen units once a day in the morning. I take an average of 40-50 units, and I know other people who take even more than that.

I asked her, "What does your doctor say about that?" She didn't want to talk about it. I watched that woman decline rather quickly and six months after her leg was amputated she died. What was her real DIS-ease, I wonder. Was she so angry that she had to live with this utterly devastating illness that she didn't even want to try to take care of herself? As I was saying, we can choose life or we can choose slow, or not so slow, death.

What I know about this woman is that she was completely overwhelmed by diabetes and she had shut down long before. She essentially died the day she was diagnosed, having not felt good about herself for some time, perhaps her whole life. It's overwhelming and catastrophic to learn you have diabetes. Then you have the business of daily and hourly control, and that can feel like a prison sentence. No wonder people get an overshadowing sense that they might as well be dead!

Stop being angry

Impatience, stubbornness, frustration, loathing, resentment, secrecy, hatred, and depression, are anger appearing in various forms. If you feel these emotions on a regular basis it is lowering your energy, making you ineffective, and keeping you a victim.

But how do you stop being angry about diabetes? How do you overcome the crushing sensation that you are now locked up for life with no possibility of parole for a crime you did not commit? Most people resign themselves to the fact and woodenly go through the motions of life. They may even be good at remembering to test three or four times a day and to count their carbohydrates. They may have concerned loved ones looking after them or looking in on them from time to time. But they have stopped participating in a life they once enjoyed.

I'm certain you are aware that bad things happen to good people. I'm sure you never intentionally set yourself up for diabetes. Who's to say why I have it and my five siblings don't? Still you have to work out your feelings about the unfairness of it all. I hear anger in response to diabetes all the time. I once told a woman with diabetes that I had it too. I was her personal coach. She said, "How can you be at all positive? How can you stand it?"

I said, "I have to take responsibility for it."

She was appalled. "What? You didn't cause it! You weren't responsible!" She was still in shock from her diagnosis and because of that she will not move forward and conquer her disease – as long as the unfairness theme is playing in her head and her emotions.

It took me a long time to realize, I am really the one who is responsible for my diabetes. It's not my dad's fault, and it's not God messing with me. It was because I happen to have a certain gene and I believe because I was on a path toward the disease for twenty years from depression and unresolved trauma (not my fault); my genes, my experiences, and my choices resulted in the symptom of diabetes. I'm not blaming myself or anyone else; not really. I am responding and listening to the message from my body. It's not the same as blaming.

And regardless of whether or not you believe you brought diabetes on yourself, the responsibility is on you from this day forward. Who is going to remind you to test? Who is going to help you resist the temptation to eat forbidden sweets and who is going to keep your blood sugar low? Who is going to do it when you don't feel like doing it? Who is going to make sure you live a happy, productive life? Everything comes down to responsibility.

Taking responsibility

If something is someone else's fault (any person or event could be to blame) I have a choice whether to allow the fault of that other person or event let *me* off the hook, or to not allow it to let me off the hook.

Here is what I mean. I may pass blame and justify not working on my DIS-ease because it's not my fault that I have it. But the problem with that kind of thinking is, whether it *was* someone or something else's fault, or not, that it was an accident of my genetics, I am the one who remains a powerless victim. When I take full responsibility, however, an amazing thing happens; I find I have the power to change my situation – to change my future.

What I told the woman was, "I take full responsibility for my life because it's my life and I am the only one who can make sure it's a happy one." And it was in that moment I had a serious *aha moment* of my own; you know the moment when you understand whatever it was you were confused about, and you get to say *aha!*

Diabetes isn't my enemy, it's my teacher.

You can begin by asking yourself, "What if this *was* my doing? How would I respond?" If you are truly honest in asking, and in taking responsibility for your diabetes, your anger will begin to diffuse and you will start to look for solutions rather than excuses.

I wish to add a little about ego here. It's your ego that's keeping you in a struggle with diabetes, as it is with any struggle. There is a piece missing when you look at what you want in your life that you are not getting. But on the other hand ego is what drives you forward to have what you want. Your ego and your high-self are two parts of you whose viewpoints are usually at odds. They are the yin and yang of you, and you need to keep them in proper balance, using your ego when it's needed, and recognizing when it's not your ego's turn to be in charge (which is most of the time). Just come to terms with your ego and don't underestimate it.

You let go of your ego by letting your deepest inner self become the part of you in charge of your life. The challenge is to allow it to happen – to get out of your own way and to stay out of your own way. It's a good, happy challenge.

How anger is hurting you

Let's dive into anger to understand how it may be hurting you. We said a little about the ego and how it controls your thoughts and emotions. You may want with all your heart to be in good control. You may have a ton of fear and worry about the devastating effects of diabetes. You may regret earlier behavior and your lack of responsibility, as I did. You may feel remorse whenever you don't do what your doctor tells you to do, whether it is counting carbohydrates, testing, exercise, or anything else she advises.

You may know it all and you may know you know what to do, and you still may not be doing it. If this describes you, you probably begin a new day, week, or month resolved to do a better job, only to find at the end of the day, week, or month it's the same old broken promises and the same familiar regret.

If you are struggling to understand your anger about diabetes, one thing will stand out: no matter how positive you try to be about it the anger is still there. One day or one moment you feel fine about the daily and hourly rituals, and sooner or later you find you are angry again. It's not difficult to be in good control when your energy is high, but when it's low the angry feelings about having diabetes just seem to take over. Those are the times when you get off track; you eat too much of something sugary or starchy, you don't feel like testing, you tell yourself you'll test later, and so on. If you're like I was, you remember to test, then remember you didn't test when you remembered, then finally test after two or three hours have gone by. This stalling is typical; it's what happens when your energy is low.

Emotions are your fuel and positive emotions give you lots of drive. Dark emotions, though, have a way of zapping your energy and leaving you drained. So when you feel bad about having diabetes, when you hate it, when you don't want to test or eat logically, it zaps your energy even more than it has already been zapped. Dark emotions spiral downward; low feelings drain energy, low energy causes you to do things contrary to good health, guilt and remorse take your energy even lower, you remember why you hate having it, and round and round you go. With diabetes we have trouble with low energy from a physiological standpoint, why make it lower with extra emotional baggage when you don't have to?

When I first learned I had diabetes I thought my life was over. I have mentioned throughout this book how angry I was and how unfair I thought it was. But one of the first things I decided to do was to get help for anxiety and depression I knew I had. I realized early on that they had factored big in why I got diabetes when I did. One of the first things I learned was I had been emotionally shut down for a long time. I was not even aware I had anger, and I had lots of it. The anger would come out sideways when my energy was low. It would come out toward my husband because he was someone safe to whom I could vent. And because he didn't have it and I did. And that seemed so unfair.

I declare that diabetes has been my greatest teacher because I began to wake up to a better way to live. I discovered on my own, like a revelation, that I could decide to not hate it instead. I could learn to let it help me become a better version of myself. And I began to come outside myself and to see a world different from the one I had perceived. I began to see a world of possibility with answers to life's problems, not just more problems. And all that from being struck with the tragedy and drama of having diabetes.

Holding On and Letting Go of Anger

Controlling anger will help you *want* to control diabetes rather than having a constant, demanding feeling that you *must* do it. This a contradiction of the type of reinforcement people usually get from well-meaning friends, family members, and doctors; the "If you don't do it then ..."

To me emotions are like three-year-old children throwing tantrums. It helps me put the whole thing into perspective and I can see how anger, over the years, has contributed to my DIS-ease.

Metaphysicians say that all illness begins with being ill at ease within the mind, or *dis-eased*. I know this is true for me; when I feel fear it's in my stomach. Stress shows up in my neck and shoulders. My body mirrors my emotions in very direct ways.

What happens after years of holding on to stress, anger, worry, and fear? Heart disease, heart attack, cancer, high blood pressure, migraines, diabetes, and more. Holding onto dark emotions shortens lives. I believe this and I'll say it again.

Holding on to dark emotions shortens lives.

And letting go is easier than you may think. As I mentioned before, when you hold onto anger, fear, or any other low emotion, you are really retaining the memory of a past feeling. In other words, emotions cannot exist in the past or future; they can only exist in the present moment. A two-year old child has curiosity about the glowing red of a stove burner until she touches it – then suddenly everything changes. She now has a bad feeling about red hot burners and she doesn't touch them again. Every time she sees one she experiences a memory of the emotions she felt from the pain she experienced when she first touched the glowing burner; she cries when she sees a red hot burner.

If you are holding on to anger you are really holding the memory of a past hurt or injustice, letting it play again in your head as though it was happening again – reliving a past moment in time. Looking at it that way, anger becomes resentment, fear becomes dread and worry, stress becomes anxiety, hatred becomes vengeance, and self-hatred becomes depression. Your brain categorizes the emotion and plays it back to you in your mind when you come to a situation that reminds you of how you felt at a earlier time. It's how we make our decisions. It's a memory that continues to teach.

This is important to understand because it is the way out of the drama and trauma of having diabetes. Did you ever notice that feelings of joy and pleasure are momentary, they don't last, and the next moment they can be gone? It's the same with anger, fear, frustration, grief, and all the other emotions you don't like feeling. If you're hanging on to them you are wallowing in past feelings. You're dredging up the past, reliving how it felt, and remaining a victim. You don't actually feel it in the moment because it became only a memory the very next moment.

Don't hold onto anger; let it go and return to a state of peace and solution-making. You probably want that instead, right? Greek mythology points to the god of the illness. In the story of Demeter, the mother of Persephone, she places a mortal child in a fire to "make him immortal." Let the illness also be the cure!

I'm not saying everyone will have an easy time letting go of their anger; some will and some won't. I am saying letting go of anger is the key to living the life you were meant to live, not in spite of having diabetes, but in concert with it, and having welcomed it into your life as part of who you are. Accept diabetes as part of who you are without letting it *define* who you are. That is the key to wellness.

People I meet, some who are powerful energy healers, tell me I am settling with having diabetes. Why would you want to *settle* when you can be healed instead? Do you believe in this miraculous type of healing? I say bring my complete healing then. I'm ready. So far it hasn't happened, though I am ready and willing for a complete healing if it is meant to be. I believe it's possible but I have yet to learn about anyone with Type 1 experiencing a complete healing. Please understand; I want a cure just as much as anyone. But I don't intend to wait for that day so I can be happy; I intend to be happy now, with or without a cure. The truth is that I consider myself healed even though I don't happen to be cured. The truth is wellness is a healthy state of mind.

The problems with fear

You may be thinking that in the case of diabetes, fear is good. Right? You would be correct. Fear of losing vision, limbs, kidney function, health, and life are power catalysts to do what the doctor says. It's what the diabetes health community is working to get you to do; *be frightened enough to change your life style.* You may want to stay in tight control due to fear that if you don't the consequences will be fatal.

So why do I say fear adversely affects blood sugar control?

Fear is a low-frequency emotion so it is limited in how much it can help you with control. In particular, *it uses a lot of precious energy.* Many people live with fear, dread, anxiety, and worry as constant companions, not even realizing they're doing it. If you live in fear, you may fear the consequences of not controlling diabetes and *still* not be doing what you need to do to improve your health and vitality.

People whose fear drives their diabetes control dread the consequences, but they usually continue to live an unhealthy lifestyle anyway, and then pile on guilt. They layer repressed anxiety with guilt, denial, and anger, and then wonder why their will-power is practically non-existent. The single biggest problem with fear when it comes to control is low energy. When our energy is low we are less inclined to do what we ought to do. We are more inclined to do what we want to do, like procrastinate, give in to temptation, and lay on the sofa.

Based upon the fear of the consequences of not doing it, medical practitioners teach people with the disease to manage and control it. In *Think and Grow Rich* Napoleon Hill discusses the six fears that hinder and stop us (Hill, 1937); poverty, criticism, ill health, loss of love from another, old age, and death. All fears can be categorized under these six. I have isolated a few of the low-vibrating emotions that accompany these fears; apathy, hatred, jealousy, guilt, anger, and sadness.

If you think about it, fear is at the core of all other low emotions. We are driven to action and inaction through fear, but fear is actually a poor way to motivate. I'm not saying fear of consequences isn't powerful, I'm just saying there is a better way. Humans are much more motivated by love, pleasure, and positive rewards.

What does it feel like when you wake up in the morning and know you need to test your glucose, count the carbohydrates in your breakfast, and do your daily exercise routine before you begin your day?

Do you love the idea? Or does it feel like drudgery? What if you could be motivated by freedom, love of life, fulfillment, and satisfaction?

I'm not claiming you would actually love diabetes management, but if you love yourself, love your life, and know why on earth you are here, it would take the sting out of having to do all those things. Testing your blood sugar, counting carbohydrates, and exercising would no longer be drudgery because these tasks would no longer be motivated by fear of failure, fear of loss of health, and fear of death. You would be motivated instead by love for yourself.

How Fear is Hurting You

Worry, anxiety, dread, distrust, entrapment, shyness, insecurity, embarrassment, doubt, caution, and tension are common forms fear takes. Fear flowing from the past is dread while fear projected into the future is worry. It's important to begin to recognize how fear has directed your thoughts and actions in the past and what you can do to keep fear from governing your future.

Like me, you may fear that life as you know it is over. I think this is true especially if you developed diabetes in adulthood, but it can be true at any age. I thought my life was over and I reacted by living a mediocre life and giving up on any dreams I once had. I didn't see that I was using fear as an excuse to live small. But fear was hurting me long before I developed diabetes; I was already living small because of fear. And fear contributed to the onset of my disease. In Chapter 1, I listed more than fifty symptoms of anxiety and depression I had. You will understand the relationship between my symptoms and my fear by looking at that list again.

You can easily see how fear of ill health would be related to diabetes, but can you also see how this fear hurts you once you have diabetes? We scare ourselves with stories we tell ourselves about what's true. There is an assumption that your health will be *ill* from this day forward and that there is nothing anybody can do to fix it. Is it true? There are diets and processes that can actually reverse Type 2 diabetes.

The story I told myself for years was that my ill health meant the end of a meaningful life for me. But developing a healthy perspective cured everything about the disease except the fact that I can't actually manufacture insulin. My new healthy perspective took the sting out of the fact of diabetes and gave me fullness in my life I had only imagined before diabetes.

If you know you're just going to die anyway from diabetes, don't you think an unhealthy perspective would stop you from pursuing your dreams? Is it true that it has to stop you?

Fear is the evil that tells us to not pursue our dreams, causes doubt about our success, and keeps us playing small. It tells us we aren't smart enough or healthy enough or sophisticated enough to succeed. But *evil* is *live* spelled backwards. Every time you become aware of some fear that's stopping you, remember it's evil. It's the opposite of living. Remember to live instead. I will help you let go of your fear.

In the third episode of *Indiana Jones*, Indy has to complete a procession of steps to obtain the Holy Grail. Eventually his steps lead to an impossibly deep chasm with no apparent way across. His instructions are related to taking a step of faith and he finally understands he has to step out into nothingness to proceed; he has to risk everything for the chance of succeeding in finding the grail. So with no other recourse he eventually steps out into the void – and immediately an invisible stone appears under his foot to support him. Hesitating again, he puts his full weight on that stone to take another step – and a bridge appears and supports him. He gets across the impossible void on those *steps of faith*.

What are you willing to risk to conquer fear? Are you open to success? How much faith do you have? Willingness to let go and trust is one of the highest attributes a person can attain. Some of us are born with it but I think it's usually learned. Once learned, though, the student becomes unstoppable.

Letting go isn't easy and conquering fear is never done quickly, so don't get hurt trying to do it all at once. Begin by letting go of something you are holding onto that seems less daunting. I began by letting go of some of my secrets – to begin to be a little more open about my experiences, to try in small ways to trust that someone else knows how I feel and wants to help me, and to start trusting myself just a little more. It builds, and little by little, you will gain more faith to take bigger steps to greater achievements that require higher risk. You let go by starting to face, rather than run from, fear.

Freefalling

Freefalling is a good word to describe letting go of fear. At the beginning of this book I told the story of my fear of success and my worry that my message isn't as important as I thought. I have been inclined to play small due to fear, a state of mind many readers will identify with. For years, having diabetes made me play much smaller than I otherwise might have done; it stopped me because I let it. It stopped me because I listened to the voice of my small-self telling me, "Your life is over."

I broke my leg while getting ready for a job interview. The voice of power and authority in my head, my *divine voice*, told me I broke my leg because I was actually and metaphorically *going in the wrong direction.* For me, it took what I would say was an act of God to change my direction. But to change my direction I needed to let go. I had to let go of my understanding of how to bring in income, I had to let go of my stubbornness about doing it my way, I had to let go of thinking it was up to me and me alone, and I had to let go of my unwillingness to trust my high ability.

I have mentored many people who went on to successfully take leaps of faith into the unknown and, having done it they've realized they were flying rather than falling. I knew the principle and how to teach it to others, and they were extremely grateful to me for helping them succeed. What I did not have was my own experience of actually taking a leap of faith that large myself. While I was helping many people it occurred to me that I had never taken the kind of leap I was helping others to do, and I realized that I didn't really want to take it. I dreaded the time when it would be required of me, and found I resisted it with all my might.

So believe me when I tell you, for anyone with or without diabetes, letting go of fear is not for the faint hearted. Like I said, my resistance was so strong it took breaking my leg to see my defiance to, and fear about, what I call *freefalling*.

Freefalling in this sense is a deeply spiritual experience. If you're as stubborn as I was I may not be able to help you change much of what you will experience with regard to freefalling, but I can save you a lot of future grief if you're open to listening.

The secret to letting go of fear is to trust yourself. Not your low self, your inner Divine self. You can call this divine part of you whatever you want; God, your super ego, your high-self, even Fred if you want. The only part of you that worries about the future, doubts your ability, and thinks you're going to die is your conscious mind, which is governed by your ego. It's difficult to believe you won't die when all the evidence in your mind and body says you will. Your mind and body know you have been dying since the day you were born; but your high-self knows the *real you* won't die, only your body dies. Your high-self trusts God, the universe, or the great unknown.

This creates conflict between the two sides of you. Your fear indicates the dying part of you is in charge while your faith indicates your divine self is running the show. We tend to move back and forth between our two minds so you can probably see that at times you have not been able to have faith and at other times you had no trouble believing, whether we're talking about faith in God, other people, or your ability to affect your circumstances. It's possible to have complete faith even when things appear to be falling apart before your eyes. What matters is which part of your mind you're listening to. How you respond to a situation depends on the strength of your faith too.

Growth's dark side

Only three per cent of us really want to know ourselves. But what you find in life to be the hardest is what you are here to learn – and it is what you will bring to the world. Nevertheless, it is the hardest. It's the shadow side of growth. Every step you take brings you closer to the light but it's the movement toward the light that causes so much pain.

My friend had a friend throughout middle school and high school. She was her best friend. Years later, a new friend came into their lives and the new friend and the old friend became best friends. After a while my friend realized the two had been telling untruths to each other about my friend until they had successfully alienated her. There are lots of reasons they did this but the point is that my friend was devastated by it; mostly because she had unknowingly allowed it by not paying attention. It kept her awake many long nights.

The hardest thing for her was letting go of the friendships with these two women that were not only not helping her, but hurting her. It was one of the toughest lessons she ever learned. But then an amazing thing happened. She looked back on it and saw she had grown tremendously. She didn't think she could survive it and when she did her confidence shot up. So when it feels like it's too hard, remember that the dark time will end; you will survive it, and you will become a better person than you were before.

The information in this chapter is important for your new code because until you begin to think differently, your various stressors will continue to do a number on your body. Add up the anger and frustration, worry, negativity, job stress, diabetes, marriage problems, unhealthy diet, unhealthy habits, smoking, trouble with relationships, inability to forgive, sleeplessness, fear, laziness, and your dogs barking at everybody who walks by your house (one of my husband's stressors), and you will come up with a number: that's the number you are doing on your body.

The emotions I have listed are the obstacles in my way of becoming worry-free, happy, and healthy. Many people manage their emotions pretty well and will need just a little help. For others, your emotions will be your biggest obstacle. You may struggle to gain control of your emotional roller coaster ride your whole life. And this battle may even be a greater battle than your battle with diabetes.

In Chapter 8 I offer you tools that have helped me gain some control of the emotional roller coaster on which I ride. Before we do that there is one more energy source to discuss.

Chapter 7. Spiritual Energy

Spiritual energy, as we described, is used up by aimlessly wandering and going in the wrong direction in life. Most people go through life in a form of unconsciousness, relying on lessons they learned in the past and solving new problems using old teachings and beliefs, without dipping into new ways of thinking.

Yes the old ways apply to your life. And the old way feels like the path to preserving energy. But when your beliefs and efforts are out of sync with *who* you are, doing something the way you've always done it actually uses more energy than finding a new, more helpful solution. That's because when you're making wrong choices, you will unconsciously give over your precious energy to the aimlessness that characterizes low energy in a spiritual sense.

The simplest way to explain this is the metaphor of driving around in a new city searching for a house, with only a vague idea and no address or map. Who would do that? It would take forever and you would become frustrated – fast. Yet people do it all the time in their aimless wandering through life.

You may be using large amounts of energy hoping if you drive around enough you will eventually run into your life's purpose. Lack of direction leaves you in a constant state of dillydallying. Most people live their entire lives not really connected to their true purpose in life, or they think they know and yet wander aimlessly. The more purposeful you are the less energy you will expend.

This is where *inspiration* comes from. When you are inspired you are "filled with the spirit" or filled with spiritual energy. Your energy seems to come from thin air. When you are inspired and taking action on the inspiration you are in such a pure spiritual state that your task requires little or no energy. You have an overabundance of energy; you feel as if you could go on forever doing whatever it is that inspires you. Most people experience this occasionally in short bursts. People living in alignment with their passion frequently feel it. Over time it can become your *natural* state.

The sad fact is, people don't know their true purpose when they don't know their value. That's the connection to energy. Someone who thinks they're worthless would logically believe God thinks they're worthless – and they would feel they have no purpose whatsoever. He or she is alive physically while dying a slow spiritual death.

If you've planned your own life and have actually followed your plan, you are in the minority. More often life happened to you, without a plan and without the proper knowledge of what you wanted or how to get it. It's not something they teach in school along-side reading and writing, but I wish it were. Within a few years you may have begun to feel as if you were off track. Then, like me, you may have decided life was good enough, or at least as good as it was ever going to get.

Most of us go through life without a plan. We may know we want to go to go to college, but not what we want to do for the rest of our lives. You may have wanted to get married and have a family because your parents did. You probably wanted to have a life to love but had no idea what your "dream" life is or how to create it. Like many, you may have thought it would show up and you would know it when it did. In the meantime, chances are you are working at a job you tolerate at best, your marriage is not what you had hoped it would be, and your friends aren't good friends.

If you're honest, you may even find yourself unhappy with your life in its current form. Why would I assume that? If you look at your friends, co-workers, and family members you will probably see a pattern of lives tossed about by the wind like the feather in the movie *Forrest*

Gump. It's the rare person who is doing what he or she absolutely loves doing and knows it's what they chose. These people are creating their lives. Life isn't just happing to them – they are the directors of it. They have power over their lives.

What are the people doing differently to be in charge of their lives? I believe it's the harder path through life – especially if, like me, you turned 18 without a clue about what you wanted. I had a vague notion that I wanted to be happy and stable and to have family and friends who loved me. But mostly I worked on surviving my rocky transition from adolescence to adulthood bridled with anger, self-recrimination, and depression, not truly believing there was anything special in store for me.

How could I have come up with a solid plan? How could I have known that I could create what I wanted to create when I didn't even know who I was? I believed that surviving was as good as it was going to ever get and it depleted every drop of my precious energy, compromised my immune system, and unknowingly stressed me out. I was not even close to figuring out I needed a plan, let alone creating one.

If you've never overcome your objections to the one life you have, you are an aimless wanderer. When you don't really like your life you don't really like yourself, since you created it to be the life you have. If you don't believe you created it you're still a victim. So the first thing to do is stop blaming other people and circumstances and simply own that you created your life to be exactly what it is.

When I owned my own life (once I got over the initial depression I had from taking responsibility for it), I began to see a way to begin to create it differently. I saw I had some actual ability to control and change my life. I was able to do it only when I finally understood exactly what I could and could not control.

I didn't have control over the circumstances of my birth or my absence of obvious talent. My brother has exceptional math ability. Two of my sisters are creative artists. My husband is a talented artist and writer and he has been passionate about the old American West since he was a child. What I was good at I thought could fit in a thimble. What I was actually good at didn't come to light until my fifties.

I often say I bought my self-esteem in my forties and I am still paying for it in college loans. Do whatever it takes. It worked. Getting an MBA shifted something huge in me. I expanded. I had new confidence which gave me the energy and capacity I needed to solve problems by giving them more focus and thought. I found enough courage to go after my dreams, and to serve, give, and appreciate others with greater fortitude, resilience, and resolve. Once that happened it took just a few more steps to find the spiritual energy source I had craved but never imagined.

I hope you can understand by this series of events how spiritual energy is killed, reborn, and revived in your life. It should give you a pretty good idea about where you are spiritually and where to go from here.

The Road to Good Health

If you love yourself you will be healthy. It's the opposite of being angry at God, your circumstances, and life. It's the opposite of victimhood. My best advice for healthy self-esteem – be who you authentically are. Even if it seems outrageous. Even if it seems impossible.

Jim Abbott isn't in the baseball hall of fame. You have probably never heard of him. He had a 10-year Major League career as a pitcher for the Los Angeles Angels and the New York Yankees where he pitched a no-hitter. He won gold at the 1988 Olympics and was a runner up for the Cy Young Award. If you have heard of Jim Abbott it's because he achieved what most of us never could, though he was born without a right hand.

Jim loved baseball so much that since the age of five he gave everything he had to learn to be a great pitcher and a better-than-average fielder and hitter – and he did all that with no right hand. Then at the ripe old age of thirty, Jim found he could no longer pitch. He had lost his fastball. He was forced to retire from baseball, the only thing with which he could truly identify. But the real story is what unfolded for him next – what I consider to be his truly authentic life. It's who he discovered himself to be after his baseball dream vanished into thin air (Abbott, 2012).

Jim's astonishing story drives home an important point, to be the person you are authentically. I mean, however outrageous it seems to you, if you trust it, it will work. I thought embracing diabetes would make me more unhappy. I could not have been more wrong. I was afraid that looking inside, at the scary mess I was inside, would be much worse than it really was. Now the most important thing I can do for my energy is to be authentic every day and to base my actions on who I am at my core. I try not to do anything that is out of alignment with me at my core. The first item in my authentic code is my spiritual care, which I define as authenticity. When I practice authenticity everything else seems to magically fall into place.

Chapter 8. It May Seem Strange at First

It's only weird if it doesn't work, Stevie Wonder says in a popular beer commercial. He was referring to Voodoo, and while this discussion is not about Voodoo, the things that work best to change what's hurting you, though seeming strange at first, really work. People tend to hold on to the negative and let go of the good. Shouldn't it be the other way around? I say, hold onto the good and let go of what's *messy*. Here are a few tools that will help you let go of what you are holding onto when you find what you are holding onto is holding you back.

Forgiveness

"Forgiveness allows us to actually let go of the pain in the memory, and if we let go of the pain in the memory, we can have the memory, but it doesn't control us. When the memory controls us, we are then puppets of the past."

~ Alexandra Asseily, *Power of Forgiveness* film

Without forgiveness people cannot move forward easily. We remain fixated on the injustice done to us. You may believe forgiveness lets the offender off the hook, but it doesn't – it lets *you* off the hook of carrying around garbage that is weighing you down and keeping you annoyed. Did you know that you can forgive someone and still be wise enough not to allow them to be around you? Forgiveness is difficult for some people.

My own grandfather preached, as though from a pulpit, that we ought not to forgive. That forgiveness is not noble. He was afraid forgiveness would let offenders off the hook. But I know that's not true. Forgiveness is a gift I give to myself. And whether you can forgive in five minutes or twenty years, I know it's worth it.

Recent scientific studies show the relationship of forgiveness to health. As many as 950 studies from 1998 to 2005 show that holding onto grudges is harmful because it disrupts breathing patterns, increases blood pressure and heart rate, and results in profuse sweating. People who are more forgiving by nature naturally have lower blood pressure and heart rate.

Dr. Kathleen Lawler-Row at East Carolina University notes that when participants in her pioneering study of forgiveness were asked to recall a troubling situation with another person, although their blood pressure went up, it resumed its normal lower rate much faster than *non-forgiving* participants (Power of Forgiveness, 2008).

Highly forgiving people have naturally lower blood pressure. However, when they talk about their personal betrayal, of the emotional moment, everyone who has been ill-treated has elevated blood pressure and heart rate. What is critical here is how long heart rates and blood pressure remain elevated. The research tells us that the longer a person remains in the agitated state the longer the vital signs remain elevated. And this is the very definition of stress.

Understand that forgiveness does not mean forgetfulness. Some people come to complete resolution while not being able to forget the offense. But through talking about it some people's blood pressure and heart rate decrease and they are quickly back to normal. Others, some of whose abuse may have been far more trivial, seem to hang on to the offenses for dear life. This slows the pattern and their vital signs remain high for longer periods, slowing recovery.

My first lesson on forgiveness was learning to forgive myself. It has been said, and I agree, that we cannot forgive others unless we first forgive ourselves. Forgive yourself (even if you don't think you need to) and forgiveness will become natural. What we know about forgiveness is that it is for the person who has been offended – for that person's health, and not for the health or happiness of the offender.

How to Let Go and Move Forward

The easiest way I've found to release emotions, including the emotions surrounding an inability to forgive, is by using a process called *The Sedona Method* (Dwoskin, 2003). It's simple, but don't let that mislead you. I quickly learned that its power is in its simplicity. This method was created by Lester Levenson and developed by Hale Dwoskin. It's a simple formula for expressing then releasing negatively charged emotions weighing you down and keeping you unhappy.

Many people, perhaps most people, hang onto troubling emotions because they do not know they can let go of them. With the Sedona method it's easy to express and then release emotions you don't want – effortlessly. You will then be able to move forward and get on with your life.

Remember, emotions only last a fleeting fraction of a second. In the next moment, when you notice you still feel the feeling, it's actually the lingering memory of what you just felt a second before. That's all. You are living in the past when you carry around a feeling you felt before; it's the *emotional baggage* psychologists refer to.

When I first began to use the Sedona Method I was skeptical. How could it be so simple? But the hardest thing about it was understanding how easy it is. It's as basic as feeling it – and then it's gone. If you find this method works for you it will help to get the book and learn all the ways to use it. I invite you to stay curious as we go through the steps. It's best to start with something less threatening until you get the idea. Then move on to bigger issues that really trouble you.

Step 1. Identify your present emotion and allow the feeling to be felt, as best you can.

Ask: *What is my "now" feeling?*

A little about the story can be helpful, but don't dwell on the story. Welcome the feeling if you can. Welcoming a difficult feeling is the most powerful way to process it, but if welcoming it is too hard to do (some things just can't be easily welcomed) use the word *allow*. Emotions are like toddlers who just want attention.

Step 2. Ask: *Could I let this feeling go?*

You are only asking yourself whether or not it's possible to let it go. "Yes" and "no" are equally valid. It's only important to be honest. Make a note of your response and go to Step 3 regardless.

Step 3. Ask: *Would I let it go?* Or *Am I willing to let it go?*

It does not matter how long it has been an issue. If you answered "no" ask, *Would I rather be feeling this or would I rather be free from it?* Move on to Step 4 regardless of your answer.

Step 4. Now ask simply: *When?*

Inviting yourself to let go right now will remind you that letting go is something over which you have complete control.

Step 5. Notice whether anything you are feeling has changed. This can range from subtle to huge. Then repeat the entire process noticing your "now" feeling. People tend to have layers of feelings buried one on top of another. The top one will come up first followed by the others in the order they have been suppressed. The first time you might feel anger. When you release it you will notice you feel a different emotion. Identify it. It may be remorse, disappointment, hatred, or something else.

The first time through the questions will be the most difficult. As you do it you will become more skilled *and* you will have less to let go. I have used the Sedona Method countless times with myself and people I work with and it has changed many lives.

If you are skeptical you are not alone. The truth is that nothing is easier than letting go of emotions, but you may have been plagued with the same feelings for years, to the point where it feels like to get out of that feeling would take a miracle. Or you may identify with the feeling like a pair of worn out slippers. You may feel as though it is impossible to let go after so long. But it *is* possible.

This method works for emotional *and* physical pain. When Hale was training our team of coaches to teach the Sedona Method he asked us to let go of trying to figure it out. I had a swollen joint in my finger for years, which became very painful at times. As he went through the questions with another woman I recognized this nagging physical pain I always had in my finger. As I asked the Sedona Method questions silently to myself (about my finger) during his demonstration I felt my own pain slip away. I still had stiffness but there was no longer any pain! Once you know this method really works you will want to use it frequently.

Limiting Beliefs

The tools above are effective for changing your state of mind and working through feelings. Now we will get to tools for changing things you actually believe to be true. Limiting beliefs can range from "Mind your P's and Q's" to "I am worthless." Where do the beliefs come from? They are memories – like recordings that constantly play in your head. So is it true?

There are many methods and processes to help you change your perspective, attitudes, thoughts, and even your beliefs. It starts with awareness, so examine what you tell yourself, and then ask yourself whether it's true. What's most important is the feeling that accompanies the thought. Identify not just how you feel – good, bad, or indifferent— but also the exact emotion you feel when you think the thought.

Think of how you feel about each of these statements. Which ones are facts? Which are beliefs? How do you feel about each belief? Good, bad, or neutral? Decide whether or not you agree with the statements. Then decide whether or not it helps you to agree with it. You may be surprised at what you learn by this exercise. Here are examples of some beliefs you can start with. If you can, start to identify yours.

The earth is round
I can't be rich
People don't like me
I am stupid
I can't control my blood sugars
I am worthless
I am smart
I am capable
I am good enough
I am not good enough
Gravity keeps me from flying off into space
I am broken
People are jerks
I'm not smart enough
I can't get a good job
Because I grew up poor I can't be rich
Because I'm over 50 no one will hire me
Happiness is overrated
Thinking about myself is selfish
I am selfish
I am not selfish
I'm not capable
Spare the rod and spoil the child
I am lazy

I should be more loving and compassionate

I should go to church more often

God loves me

God does not love me

I should think more about other people

What is the matter with me?

I hate _____ (fill in the blank)

Mom likes my sister better than me

I don't deserve it

I love God

Mom loves my sister more than me

I hate testing my blood sugar

I hate having to be in control of this disease

I am not in control of my health

I can't have good control *and* be happy

I never have anything clever to say

It's _____'s fault

I never fit in

I'm not lovable

I'm weak

I shouldn't be mad at God

I hate diabetes

I never know how much insulin to take

I love dogs

I am special

I have rare gifts

I hate myself

I am ugly

I am fat

I am not good at anything

I hate liver

I am not creative

There is nothing special about me

For some of these beliefs there is enough evidence to support believing them. Other examples will not apply to you. And some of them will hit home. I believe the earth is round and there is much evidence to support that belief, so I keep it. I once believed I was useless but I really had no evidence to support it. People I love told me it wasn't true but I still believed it. The purpose of the list is to help you start to identify the things you say to yourself so you can decide for yourself how you really feel, whether a belief is true or just true to you, and what you want to tell yourself instead. Start identifying some of your beliefs right now so you can begin to change the ones you want to change.

Take a blank sheet of paper and make two columns. On the left side list your beliefs and put a check next to the beliefs you feel are not helping you, or worse, are even hurting you. It's not necessary to include physical categories on your list like the ones I have listed. It's what you believe about yourself and other people, God, and life that may be hurting you.

Affirmations

In the right column, next to the statements on your list you know are hurting you, create statements that say what you want to believe instead. If you have trouble, remember it's just the opposite of what you recognized you are currently saying. So my belief *I am useless* becomes *I am useful*. When you turn the statement around use only positive words. This is the most challenging part. Don't write *I am not useless* or *I am not weak* (say I am strong), etc.

The simplest way to change beliefs you do not want to support is to take away their power. They had no power to begin with; they are simply things you believed long ago, perhaps since your childhood, which probably served you then. Now, however, some of those beliefs that served you when you were younger may be causing you problems. And the best thing you can do in that case is choose to believe something else instead.

I had a belief that God is vengeful and I had better go to church and behave as a good Christian should, or I might go to hell. To me it was a fact. I had to move on from that belief and I did it by challenging it. It was not easy – changing my spiritual beliefs has been more difficult than changing any of my other beliefs. Spiritual beliefs go right to your core. And challenging them felt like blasphemy to me.

Beliefs about yourself, that you're not likeable or you don't fit in, are difficult because they seem to come from your very core, too. When I started working on my beliefs about myself I was able to change some of them because it made logical sense; I understood that I came from the same place everyone else came from. My belief that I was somehow less than other people, *I'm not lovable,* was based on a belief I had held since childhood that simply was not logical. I changed how I perceived myself by forming new habits – forming new neural pathways in my brain from new habits that said the things I wanted to believe about myself instead.

Relentlessly, several times a day, whenever I became aware of a negative thought about myself, or a low feeling I felt that identified something I thought, I consciously and purposefully said *STOP!* to that thought and replaced it with the new thought. Then just to be sure, I repeated the new thought like a chant so it would begin to run unconsciously, like a recording. At first I had a lot of trouble. The hardest part was that as soon as I began the work I saw how much of an uphill battle it would be. There were so many. I had had no idea how many there were and how many of my hours were spent listening to those damaging tapes that played over and over.

It took me about two months of aggressive work on my personal beliefs (by identifying them as merely habits that needed changing), and then I had an incredible dream where I was in control of my life and I knew I was transformed. It wasn't impossible, it didn't take forever, and while difficult, I don't remember the pain now, I just appreciate the permanence of the change and my new authentic self that emerged from all the turmoil.

Since my experience with positive affirmations, which always work but take a lot of constant effort, I have found a very interesting process for changing beliefs and when I use it my inner thoughts and feelings seem to automatically support the change, making it much less work. And I never cease to be amazed at how easy it is.

Changing Your Beliefs Effortlessly

The methods discussed here are stress management techniques that are easily and quickly mastered by many people. They are not intended to take the place of psychotherapy. People who have medical or emotional problems that require professional attention should use these programs as they would any other stress relief method, and under the supervision of a physician or other qualified health professional.

Of the methods I have used to actually change my perspective PSYCH-K® (Williams, 2009) is my very favorite. This process will change what you believe to be true, whether the belief is consciously or subconsciously held. At first I wanted to use it to change my belief from *I can't heal from diabetes* to *I can heal*. What happened next, while it did not change that belief, showed me where to begin.

While there are many processes for healing, changing beliefs, and changing energy, this one seems to have found me. That's because it was a *vibrational match* for me. This is a process for changing beliefs to match what you want to believe or even beliefs that you already *think you believe*. That is, you may already believe it; the surprise comes when you learn you really don't believe it – not completely, and you realize that's why you have not had the success, health, wealth, happiness, and the relationships you desire.

Using PSYCH-K® I changed my beliefs about my relationship with God and at least 20 limiting beliefs about my relationship with myself and with my challenging illness. And when I did, something shifted every time. Maybe not immediately, and never in the same way, but a burden always lifted and my perspective changed for good.

I thought I could change my belief that I cannot heal my illness. What I found I really needed to change were my beliefs about my higher power and my higher ability. Then after I completed those changes I began to understand how important it is to believe I am important to God, and I changed my belief from *God doesn't even know I'm here,* to *I am important to God ... I am an expression of God.*

I found real power when I realized I didn't believe it or I didn't want to believe it anymore and then actually changed the belief. We often surprise ourselves when we understand we have been operating from a completely different reference point than what we thought.

My new path took me from hating my illness to having no anger – yes, especially when I think about it. I began to take care of it no differently than remembering to make my bed or water my plants. I took the edge off my disease.

The Process:

We begin by muscle-testing a belief. Every cell in your body vibrates with the energy of everything you know. Every cell "knows" what your conscious mind has filtered out as unimportant. That means when you need to make a decision it would be helpful to ask your body, don't you think? We know far more at the subconscious level than at the conscious level. That means your cells are in some ways more intelligent than your conscious mind. In fact, our consciousness usually interferes with discovering valuable truths about ourselves.

But the muscles and organs of our bodies have all our subconscious truth and our muscles can reveal it using a simple, reliable binary code. Chiropractors, holistic clinics, massage therapists, and energy healers use muscle testing extensively to get to the core of disease and DIS-ease that weighs on people. With this process it is used solely for testing subconscious beliefs and for the Balancing process protocols.

Every muscle in your body can be muscle-tested so muscle-testing can be done a number of ways. Remember, your cells *know* all your true beliefs, and that means your muscle cells *know* them. In a nutshell, when the muscle is strong your belief statement is true; when it's weak and you can't hold it strong, it's false. When I test someone's muscle with the statement "I have high confidence" and they can't hold their muscle strong, no matter what they say about their confidence I know it's low.

The belief that came up for me to change first, the one that wasn't *healing from diabetes*, was that I was *disconnected from my source*. The moment that statement was read to me I knew it was not only true, but also my most limiting belief; if you remember, at that time I was not certain I believed in a higher power. We muscle tested and, sure enough; I could not hold my arm strong. We did what is referred to as a *PSYCH-K® Balance* and I felt a big shift. Afterward my muscle tested strong and for the next month I began to notice a shift in my spiritual thinking – to thoughts, feelings, and actions that supported a solid belief in God – a belief that has been with me ever since.

After that experience I worked on finding out what I needed to change next. Here are some of the belief changes I have made to date using PSYCH-K®. I use the term *God* in my practice but use the term for your Source or Higher Power that is right for you. The chart says all that needs to be said about this incredible process. As you will see in Part Three this was the beginning of my authentic diabetes code.

Old Belief	New Belief	The Learning
God, if He exists, does not matter to me	God is important to me	Continuously renewed spiritually, on a spiritual journey, continually in touch with God
God could not possibly think about me	I am important to God	God loves me; I am a physical expression of God.
I can't live the life I want if I want good diabetes control	I can have good diabetes control *and* live the life I want	The only thought in the way was my own belief about what is possible
I hate diabetes	Diabetes is an important part of who I am	If not for diabetes I would not be who I am today
I don't want to take care of diabetes	I want to take care of diabetes	I care about myself enough to take care of myself
I can't control diabetes	I control diabetes	HA1c results consistently in the sixes
Having diabetes is hard	Diabetes is easy	When I think about it now there is no drama or anxiety
I never want to test so I do not test when I remember to	I automatically test when I am reminded by a thought to test	It hurts about as much as putting on makeup
I forget to test	I remind myself every time it's time to test	My intuition, when I listen, picks up when I fail to remember

Old Belief	New Belief	The Learning
My blood sugars are always high in the morning	My blood sugars are normal in the morning	Morning blood sugar levels consistently 80-120
I don't know how much to dose	I intuitively know how much to dose every time	When I need to guess my inner guide tells me
I don't have a good system to help me with diabetes	I have a great system for treating and tracking diabetes	My ideal authentic code showed up immediately after I started changing my approach
I constantly crave sweets and carbohydrates	I don't crave sweets and carbohydrates	I am more consistent. I lost 30 lbs. without even trying

It's important to remember that results will vary. The process can sometimes create a strong emotion, depending on the issue. For me, for the next few weeks after my muscle tests strong for a new belief, I begin to notice a shift in my thinking – to thoughts that support my new belief. Then I find I am able make easier and faster progress.

PSYCH-K® requires a systematic approach to beliefs and it has been organized in such a way as to make it safe and, for lack of a more precise word, permissible. You would not want to change a belief unless it was in your best interest, so we use muscle-testing to find the first belief to change, according to your higher self, then we ask your subconscious self for support and permission to change it. For this reason it's important to hire a PSYCH-K® facilitator trained to understand what is going on. Contact me for more information. My contact information is at the back of the book.

Don't suffer needlessly. Is there suffering in the world? Yes. Will you suffer from something in the future? Probably. The point is, we suffer well beyond when the time to suffer is over and the time to live has come. I am certain it's usually caused by beliefs we hold on to that limit us. With each limiting belief you change you will move forward faster and easier.

Meridian Tapping

Tapping on your acupuncture points can help alleviate stress and anxiety caused by whatever you are thinking about at the time. This technique works wonders for phobias. For people with diabetes it can help calm you enough to gain perspective and using it to intervene can eliminate destructive behaviors like giving in to cravings; if you crave sugar, use a pre-determined tapping process and feel your craving slip away like magic.

Tapping takes advantage of the tendency all humans have to use our hands to comfort ourselves; we naturally make contact with the comfort spots on our bodies with our hands. Many of the traditional acupuncture points are in fact such comfort spots, however, rather than using invasive needles, tapping uses a gentle and reassuring form of touch. With this simple system you can easily master it to use on yourself *and* teach it to others.

For maximum effect:

Have a pen and paper handy as you go through the basic instructions. You will tap on the eight comfort spots in the following sequence:

1. Karate Chop Spot: Halfway between the wrist and the base of the little finger on the outside of either hand. It's the part a Karate master uses to split a board in two.

2. Inner eyebrow Spot: At the inner corner of either eyebrow next to the bridge of the nose.

3. Outer-eye Spot: At the outer corner of either eye on the bone.

4. Under-eye Spot: Just beneath either eye in the middle on the bone.

5. Under Nose Spot: Directly beneath the nose.

6. Under Mouth Spot: Directly under the mouth.

7. Collarbone Spot: Make a fist and lightly thump the two upward pointing bones just beneath your throat below the area called the Adam's apple.

8. Under Arm Spot: About four inches under the armpit on either side. Use the full hand to tap this spot.

9. Top of Head Spot: Toward the front.

Step 1. Measure your stress level. On a scale of 1-10 determine your stress level with 10 being as upset as you can possibly be and 0 being completely unbothered. Write down the first number that comes to you.

Step 2. Choose an issue following these guidelines: a memory that troubles you and that you don't want, with an intensity of 5 or higher at the moment, but not a 9 or 10. Choose a specific scene that represents the issue for you in its most upsetting and most vivid sense.

Step 3. Recall the scene with great detail.

Step 4. Create a mental movie with beginning and end to help you assign the intensity rating.

Step 5. Take an intensity rating and write the number down. Choose the first number that comes to mind.

Step 6. Create a title for it to remind you and write down the title.

Step 7. Create a statement that begins with "Even though…" followed by a statement of the problem and a positive, affirming statement that tells you how you would like to feel instead, like "… I choose to be calm and confident." Your statement might be something like, "Even though I feel nervous speaking to large crowds, I choose to be calm and confident."

Step 8. Create a reminder phrase to help you remember, similar to your title.

Step 9. Prepare by tapping the Karate Chop spot lightly but vigorously while saying the entire tapping statement three times out loud.

Step 10. Proceed through the 9 steps, tapping lightly but vigorously at each spot.

Now rate the intensity of the issue again. Modify your tapping statement to reflect the changing emotions around the issue. It may change from feel sad to feel a little sad, etc. End the tapping session when the rating has decreased to a "2" or lower on all the feelings surrounding the issue. If you are unable to reach this level there is likely another aspect of it you need to address (Carrington, 2008).

When I learned tapping, the instructor had each of us think about a situation that scares us. For some it was flying in an airplane or standing on the roof of a sky scraper. What used to scare me most was speaking to a large crowd. When I pictured myself in front of a group of 500 it would trigger so much anxiety I was in physical pain.

The instructor led us through the tapping technique while we each imagined our scary situation. What impressed me was that, while I really did notice no more butterflies when I thought about speaking to a large crowd, I also didn't feel any anxiety when I thought about speaking to even 5000, on any subject, with little or no advance preparation. And all I had done was take a risk and try a method called *Tapping*.

Healing Yourself

A note about *energy* medicine. Five thousand years ago humans had a much different take on healing and medicine. The medicine man or woman, called a shaman, sought to understand the underlying cause of an illness. He or she would get to the root of the problem using energy medicine. They did not just treat the symptoms, as is generally the case with modern allopathic medicine. While today's medicine men and women can help you manage diabetes they usually cannot cure you with their techniques.

Ancient Hindu medicine people recognized seven major energy centers and 20 minor ones in and about the human body. Energy healers access these centers to understand the real cause of an illness in order to cure it. The word chakra is Sanskrit for "wheel" or turning. When your chakras are spinning or turning correctly your body corresponds with good health. When they are stuck or turning in the wrong direction you have symptoms.

The third chakra, the solar plexus chakra, is the seat of power and identity. I do not profess to be a shaman but I am certain this was my original problem – the one that brought on my DIS-ease. Powerlessness. The third chakra is located in the lower abdomen, right where the pancreas sits. Consult the resources section at the back of the book to begin to learn more and find healing for your energy (King, 2011).

You will use many processes and methods on your journey through life. Identify whether you want to explore some of the tools I have given you. You may know of others as well. What you do will depend largely on what you like since the ones you use will most likely choose you.

Part 3. Your Authentic Code

Chapter 9. Principles to Help You Get Ready

I didn't set a goal to develop my new code. It was my unsuccessful experience with the insulin pump that led me to my ideal system. When I found I could not use the pump it didn't devastate me as it would have just a couple of years before. That was because I had healed my DIS-ease – the things about me that caused extreme frustration with diabetes. Instead I decided there must be a better solution for me and I set about to find it.

Most people will live their lives not accomplishing their goals or realizing their true potential. We are more powerful than we know, yet we are more vulnerable than we want to admit. I have learned through much trial and error what works for me to achieve big things, and while I could do better on much of it, I do have a map now and it has made a huge difference in achieving big goals. It makes it easier and quicker. If accomplishing something is difficult you can see why some of your heart's desires have not been achieved.

The most important aspect of achieving big goals is that you must have enough drive and forward momentum. I refer to it as your WHY. Some people come into this world with enough ambition and motivation to accomplish just about anything they set their minds to. They are the exception and I doubt many of them are reading this. For the rest of us, to give you enough energy when it gets tough, connect the *big goal* you want to achieve with something you feel passion about *at your core*. Something you love. The way to tie your new diabetes code to your core desire is by being the top priority to yourself.

Here is one example: *I want to learn to cook Tai food*, might be a big goal for someone who loves cooking, but not for someone who doesn't like to cook. Tying it to what you love will give you enough energy and drive to actually achieve it. And achieving a big goal such as learning to cook Tai food will actually do much more for you than just achieving that one goal. When you are successful at something you didn't think you could do you find your confidence has increased and you have changed in bigger ways than you would have thought.

Before you get started developing your code I would like to give you the most important guidance principles for achieving any big goal. Bookmark this section and return to it when you feel lost, frustrated, or stuck.

1. Take a few minutes to write down your big goal. Tape it to your computer screen, on the mirror, or in some other prominent place. Look at your goal every day and think about what you are going to do today to accomplish it. With the goal front and center in your mind you will continuously work to achieve it. For this process I recommend a goal of: Develop a personalized system for managing my diabetes that gives me energy and the life I want (or something similar).

2. Make a declaration. Garrett Gunderson, one of my mentors and the author of a best-selling book about gaining control of your money, decided he was going to do a triathlon competition. He grew a beard and let his hair grow. For the next three months he conducted all his business unshaven and long-haired. He is a public speaker and fastidious about his appearance, so appearing on stage that way had a huge effect on him as well as on others. Every time he spoke on stage he declared,

"I'm going to do a triathlon and I'm not going to shave or cut my hair until I do it. I want everyone in this room to hold me accountable to finish."

He succeeded! That kind of dedication to a goal makes it nearly impossible to fail (Gunderson, 2009).

3. Breathe and relax. How do you eat an elephant? One-bite-at-a-time. No one ever accomplished a big goal by doing everything at once, and yet that's what people try to do. Give yourself a break instead.

Once you begin the process of accomplishing your goal you will start to see progress; small at first, but enough to motivate you to keep going. If you want to be successful at anything you have to be patient and remember to stay calm. I look at it like the Titanic – you know, huge ship, tiny rudder? We have tiny rudders, so to speak, and you are trying to turn around a gigantic ship built from all the beliefs you have accumulated over a lifetime.

As long as you keep moving forward you will make better progress than you did the day before, but no matter how much you work on it every day it's going to take time to turn a ship like that around. On the bright side, once it's turned it will stay – turned.

4. With me – without me. Whether you hire an expert or recruit a friend, having someone else to help you face your wall will be the difference between conquering it and running away. You need to get outside your comfort zone and having someone there holding your hand helps. In many cases it is the difference between success and failure!

People hesitate to hire a coach because they don't know the value. Whether or not you know your coach, and whether or not you are paying her, if the person coaching you isn't helping you, you will not believe coaching helps much. So if your coach is not helping you change your life, get a new coach.

The changes you will be able to make by having a good coach will be much deeper than trying to change on your own. By having someone hold your hand you will be more open to going deep – where real change can occur. I made progress until I had my first breakthrough about twenty years later – without a mentor. I thought I was doing just fine and I guess in a way I was. But I experienced my second major breakthrough in less than three months. I make much faster progress when I have mentors. To keep you from running away from your troubles get someone to help you.

5. Become your own coach. Good coaches coach by listening, being objective, and encouraging their students. The natural next step is to become good at coaching yourself.

As much as I help people as their coach I always maintain that you are your true coach. Your coach has guided you to where you are right now; your intuition led you to your first job, your sweetheart, your career, and everything else you have wanted and received. As your own coach you will begin to base everything you do on honesty. Have you ever felt inspired to be truly authentic, and then everything came beautifully together?

Have you ever second-guessed your original thoughts, changed your mind, and then things fell apart? We sabotage ourselves when we second-guess our intuition. Perhaps you don't believe in your abilities. Or you may be a perfectionist, which leads to second-guessing your original decision, which leads you to make unwise choices, which keeps your confidence low. You may make a decision, then doubt the decision, and then make the wrong choice instead. I used to do this regularly. Be aware of the tricks you use to sabotage yourself.

Use your inner GPS. Gather tools that will help you go deep; ask difficult questions you tend to resist asking. Do things you have resisted in ways you have resisted doing them. This is self-coaching.

6. Keep track of your milestones. You know you have made a breakthrough if you know you would never go back to your old ways. It's your job to hold yourself accountable and your breakthroughs will help do that. Without breakthroughs you will not continue this program of creating your ideal system. You will give up. By looking at your progress you will be able to keep going when things get tough.

7. Embrace the dark side of your goal. Fear, doubt, and anxiety are all part of accomplishing anything big. When you feel dark or negative feelings, remember that they are a necessary part of achieving your goal. Everyone who ever accomplished something big did it while feeling fear and doing it anyway. Bravery is not the absence of fear – it's doing big things in spite of how you feel. Failure reinforces growth. Don't worry if you feel like you are failing. You may tell yourself you can't do something because of some previous "failure." Success is great, but honestly, we learn much more from our failures than from our successes. We learn even more from embracing the dark side of a goal than from accomplishing the goal. It's true.

8. Commit, commit, commit. Before you begin you must make a firm commitment to stay committed no matter what. If you cannot commit you will not succeed. And remember, the very best way to build your confidence is to keep the promises you make to yourself. When you don't keep the commitments you make to yourself it carves away your self-esteem – just like a fast river does to its bank. But when you keep the promises you make to yourself you will achieve not only your goal, but also more self-confidence, greater authenticity, and higher energy.

9. Be important to yourself. Be as important to yourself as other people are important to you. Without this you will put yourself and your work lower on the priority list and get the same old frustrating outcomes. Being important to yourself makes logical sense too; how could anyone else be any more important than you?

10. Use your imagination. The greatest triumphs are achieved with imagination. Creativity and imagination are accessed through your intuition. But you have to trust yourself to be able to listen to and *trust* your intuition. The best way to access your imagination is to have confidence in yourself. The more confident you become the more imaginative you will be able to be.

You imagination will help you become clear about your goal, create your plan for achieving it, solve problems as they arise, stay motivated, have energy, and succeed in a way you could not have imagined before you called on your imagination to help you achieve it.

Many people go about their lives closed to possibilities and unaware that's what they are doing. We tend to go through life in survival mode, taking care of physical needs and ignoring our emotional, spiritual, and soulful needs, which are necessary for a happy and successful life.

Chapter 10. The Grit: Discovering Your Diabetes Programming

Even a person with eyes will be able to see an object in darkness only with the help of a lamp.

~ Ancient Sanskrit Proverb

Steps for Creating Your System

I am now going to give you a series of tools to use in developing your code. You will use them at different times and for different things; you may use them for the rest of your life. As you go through this process please refer back to various sections of the book to help you. For instance, include objectives that will help with each of the four types of energy: physical, mental, emotional, and spiritual. The personality key motivators discussed in Chapter 2 can help you identify the elements of your unique code.

For purposes of this program I have listed the steps I took to develop my code. You may find you want to use a different order, however. There were essentially eight steps I had to take to get to where I am today, free from the suffering that inherently comes with diabetes.

Step 1. Remember what you experienced when you were diagnosed

Step 2. List the things that are not right in your life

Step 3. Identify the problem at the core

Step 4. Begin work to heal the core DIS-ease

Step 5. Identify your limiting beliefs one by one

Step 6. Change your limiting beliefs

Step 7. Write your new Authentic Diabetes Code

Step 8. Support your new code every day

Worksheets

First you need to understand how you feel about all the issues we have discussed regarding the physical, mental, emotional, and spiritual aspects of diabetes. I recommend you complete the worksheets to get a measurement of your temperature when it comes to diabetes. Be as specific as possible. The more specific you are, the better you will understand what you need to do to fix your current broken system. It all begins with honesty with the self. Be completely honest or don't waste your time. Be as nurturing with yourself as possible as you complete the worksheets on the following pages.

Keeping tabs daily will give you a good idea about your current code. Make copies of Worksheet 2 or simply record your thoughts and feelings each day in a journal for a week. You will want to keep the notes handy for reference. Once you have done that you will begin to have a pretty good idea about what you need to work on first.

Complete the worksheets and we will discuss the eight steps in more detail.

Worksheet 1 Do this once then keep it handy for reference
How do you deal with anger, grief, exhaustion, fear, or other energy zappers without causing your blood sugar to increase? Use details
Do you feel guilty after a high blood sugar result? What do you do about it?
What aspects of your emotional and mental state of mind do you think are affecting your glucose levels? Start by thinking of one obvious one. Others will come to mind. List them as they come up. As you think of more come back to this page to record them.
Do you agree or disagree with how your doctor is helping you treat diabetes? What would you change about your current treatment? What would you like to add if you could?
a) What issues from your past continue to play again and again in your mind? b) What are you doing about it?

Do you know if you have depression and/or anxiety? Is it chronic? Go into detail if you can.
On a scale of 1-10 rate your feelings about having diabetes. 1 = hate it, 10 = no problem (11 = love it)
What system do you use for monitoring your blood sugar? Examples: insulin pump, glucose meter, blood glucose logs, etc. How often do you test? What readings do you consider ideal? What do you consider too high? Too low? What problems do you typically have with controlling diabetes?
On a scale of 1 – 10 rate your feelings about blood sugar monitoring: 1 = you despise it. 10 = it's not a problem.
What was your last HA1c?
Estimate your average HA1c for the past 1-2 years

What tools do you use to regulate and monitor your diet? Examples: carbohydrate calculator, insulin pump, recipes, diet foods, a regimented diet, etc. List all your tools
What tools or methods do you use or want to try for management of your thoughts, beliefs, and feelings? List them here
Do you have a supportive family or friends, a support group, or do you chat about diabetes in an online forum? Discuss
On a scale of 1 – 10 how satisfied are you with your level of control?
On a scale of 1 – 10 how satisfied are you with your quality of life?
On a scale of 1 – 10 rate your self-esteem
What are your beliefs about yourself and your role on earth? Discuss

Worksheet 2 Make several blank copies of this worksheet. Do this exercise daily for at least one week or until you have a good idea about what is going on. Your answers will vary from day to day.

What is your blood sugar average today?

Take your current mental and emotional temperature. Rate yourself on a scale of 1 – 10, 1 = you hate yourself and you want to stay in bed, 10 = you're ready for anything. Write about it

Are you sad or depressed today? If so write about it.

What issues from your past have been playing in your mind today? Thoughts *and* feelings

What have you learned today about what you need to start to do?

What are you going to do today to develop your ideal code?
On a scale of 1-10 rate your level of control today.
On a scale of 1 – 10 rate your satisfaction with your level of control today.
On a scale of 1 – 10 rate your level of happiness today.
On a scale of 1-10 rate your level of self-esteem today. 1 = It's in the toilet, 10 = I'm king/queen of the hill.

Begin to write your code by indicating on this chart your current problems and possible solutions . We will work on better solutions later – once you have established what needs fixing.

Your Diabetes Code

Use my code as a template. Remember; you may have completely different issues than I had.

Current problem	Your current code	Your authentic code	Note
		(add this later)	

Current problem	Your current code	Your authentic code	Note

Belief Change Worksheet

Use this form to identify beliefs you want to change, formulate your new beliefs, and record your results. Many of your beliefs and most of your results will show up later so don't worry about completing it yet. Feel free to use any of my beliefs if you find you have them, too. They are listed in a Table in Chapter 8 (page 141).

Old Belief	New Belief	The Learning

The Steps

It's OK if you read through the entire book before you really dive in. But start now to identify the problems and record them as you think of them. I had no worksheets, questions, or tools when I created my diabetes code. I have designed the worksheets based on what I intuitively did as I developed my code. At each step the specific tasks will help you become clearer. Or you may choose to take a more organic approach and just use some of my ideas to create your ideal system yourself.

Step 1 What you experienced when you were diagnosed

As best you can, make a record of the following. This will help you understand your personality, a key feature in developing your code. It may also hold clues to some of your limiting beliefs, which will be important. At the end of this tour through the steps I have summarized them, along with when to use all the tools, questions, and worksheets.

Tell the story of the experiences that led to your diagnosis.

I was newly married and had a young son only one and a half years old. I worked full-time at a state job that was the most stressful position I have ever held. It was April of 1985 and something wasn't right. I had always been pretty healthy and had only a few minor health complaints.

But this was serious. I started to lose weight for no reason. I was thirsty all of the time and I craved sugary sweets. But I was losing weight, not gaining. Then I became extremely constipated and my vision started getting blurry. I have to admit it took me several weeks to see a doctor. He knew it immediately the instant I told him my symptoms. When he tested my blood sugar it was over 700.

The doctor I saw kept it clinical. He prescribed some pills to begin with but I think he knew they weren't going to be enough – that I had Type 1 diabetes.

What did you feel?

I went home and sat on my bed and cried. My husband came home with our son a while later. My toddler tried hard to console me. It felt the way I feel when someone close to me has died. It felt like when my mother died. In a way it felt like I had died.

What did you think about?

I thought, hoped, that the drugs would work and I wouldn't have to go on shots. But I knew I probably had Type 1 like my father. I thought about going to talk with my father. I thought about how we had been talking about having another baby and now this would change everything. I thought about my stressful job and all the other stress I had been under. Our apartment had been burglarized just a few weeks earlier.

Step 2 List the things that are not right in your life

Begin to identify things that were not right in your life and health at the time. Start with a list.

My list did not immediately come to me. This part really took a long time to complete. As I said before, let's hope yours can come together much faster but it takes as long as it takes so be patient. Having my tools and my experience should speed it up for you. This is not a list for finding fault; it is to help you understand your current situation.

1. Stressful job and lack of realistic stress-relief techniques

2. Chronic sinus infections for years from a broken nose in childhood *and* chronic allergies
3. Childhood abuse resulting in Depression/Anxiety Disorder that went undiagnosed and untreated for two decades
4. Untreated low self-esteem and lack of a healthy identity

Step 3 Identify which problem is at the core

It took three years but I finally understood that my self-esteem was in the toilet and I didn't really know who I was or what I was doing with my life. This was a huge insight and it took me a long time to realize it because all my life I had pretended to myself (and the world) that I knew who I was and liked who I was. The truth didn't just come to me one day either – it had to unfold slowly and painfully until one day I hit on it – my real DIS-ease was that I didn't like myself, didn't think I was very likeable (I wasn't back then), and didn't think God could possibly like me either. BINGO!

Don't stop until you hit BINGO. The solar plexus chakra is the seat of our power and identity. I didn't know about chakras when I started learning to like myself though. I just knew not being in charge of my life was ruining my life and that it had likely brought on diabetes.

I think diabetes almost always has to do with a problem with personal power stemming from something in a person's life, whether it was from abuse, some other traumatic experience, your response to an event or situation, or your personality. The severity of the event or issues doesn't seem to be as important as the severity of your response to it. It could have been immediate or gradual, as a child or as an adult. Unresolved power-issues come out sideways, so to speak; these issues are lodged and stored in your body and often (always?) show up as symptoms of some illness.

If you don't like yourself and/or don't develop your own sense of who you are, you are giving away your power, a very dangerous activity. I'm not saying you will get diabetes, but I think it's why a lot of people have it.

Step 4 Begin work to heal your core DIS-ease

I worked on my self-esteem for the next five years, and slowly but continually after that. I went to college in my thirties, something I had never worked up the courage to tell my husband I wanted to do.

Work on everything on your list but focus most importantly on that one core problem you identified. If you were not able to identify the core problem you are not in touch with yourself. People who want to go and find themselves are delusional. There is no *finding yourself.* You have been *right here* all along. The actual problem is with not wanting to take a real look. Seek the core issue until you find it. That's all I can say about it.

Before we go into the next step I am going to talk in more detail about low self-esteem. If you think your self-esteem is high feel free to skip this part. But I believe low self-esteem is a world-wide scourge. It's nothing to be ashamed of or embarrassed about but shame and embarrassment are the reason it's such a problem – people just don't want to admit it. To me it's only one of the costs of being human. I have said that humans are the only creatures who remember failure and continue to punish themselves and each other over and over again for that failure.

In Chapter 1 we talked about how to identify low self-esteem. Please go back to page 15 and ask yourself those questions again. I think it's true for everyone that the hardest blow your ego can take is realizing you don't like yourself. It was true for me and also for hundreds of other people I know. We will believe almost anything rather than admit it. Learn muscle testing and if you think your self-esteem is fine you will be able to test it for yourself.

We lie to ourselves and we lie to other people, but it's the truth that will set you free. "My self-esteem is fine," is a lie many people tell themselves. It *is* the DIS-ease! Think about it. Does a child naturally love himself? As an infant, yes. And a loving parent who values herself will work hard to continue to instill it in her child because self-esteem is fragile and can very easily be taken away. But what if a mother or father has no idea of her or his own value? How can these parents teach self-value to their children? And we've seen what really happens – too often they unknowingly teach the child he has little or no value.

Parents have an even more difficult job because teachers, peers, friends, bullies, and even strangers (guilty and innocent), tell children they aren't loveable, likeable, smart, capable, or cute enough. Too often the world teaches children they aren't good enough. So even when parents have high self-esteem they have a huge job deliberately instilling self-value in their kids at every step along the treacherous path to adulthood.

So while eighty-five per cent of kindergarten children have healthy self-esteem only twenty per cent do at high school graduation (Canfield). It's a scourge and you're not doing yourself a favor pretending you have a healthy sense of *who you are* if you don't. The reason I say healthy self-esteem is so important for people with diabetes is that I think it is often at the core of all the trouble – low self-value. Being truthful about where you are right now is the beginning of learning to like yourself. If you are able to be honest you will actually begin to like yourself – even love yourself. In time you will be so tickled to be you that you will hardly be able to stand it!

Self-esteem is not just about liking yourself. It may be true that you like yourself fine and have diabetes. If so, you have an advantage. However, you still may not know why the heck you're here on Earth. And you still may be giving away your power.

Identify for yourself what you need to start working on and get to work on it. No matter what, focus on healing the core DIS-ease that caused you to develop the symptom of diabetes. This sickness at your core has to be the WHY of doing this work or you will stop working on it. The ability to face and not run from whatever it is you need to begin working on, which will be a very scary thing, is the secret to developing your code. Remember, it's not easy, but it's worth it. And believe me it's only hard at first. All the work is up front. Then it's smooth sailing.

I have told you where to begin if you identify a lack of self-value and I know what to do if your identity is the problem – you know, the feeling that you are glad you're here but you don't know *why* you're here. This "lack of self-value" could be from some other core problem. I don't know what it is but you do – at your core. And when you search for it you will find it.

In my case there were other issues as well, and I was able to address them. For my stressful job, being *aware* did a lot to help me alleviate much of the stress associated with the job. Learning stress relief techniques, taking regular breaks, and starting to care more about myself helped even more. I didn't know it but looking back I wasn't taking care of myself because I didn't think I mattered. It wasn't a conscious choice, but that choice affected everything.

Begin to do things you have not been doing, whether it's caring more about you, dealing with your stressors, gaining more knowledge, having conversations with people, or meditating and journaling to help you discover what it is you need to start doing differently.

Step 5 Identify you're limiting beliefs one by one

I didn't think I believed in God any more. At first I thought the problem was that I didn't believe I could heal from diabetes. I was very surprised to find that my core limiting belief was about my spirituality. I knew immediately that it was a big problem, although I didn't know how it was connected to healing from diabetes.

In my teens I joined a Christian group and became *born again* as they say. When I accepted Jesus I thought my problems were over. I was able to move out of my parents' home without going on the run. The group I found loved me and taught love and respect. They were a true family; the family I had been missing. While in that group I learned who Jesus is. I read the Bible every day and I learned about repentance and forgiveness. It helped. I stayed with that religious group for five years.

But although the experience helped me I still did not think much of myself. I didn't know I thought so little of myself and I surely didn't know what a big problem it was. It was my central problem! My religion taught that the Bible teaches us not to think highly of ourselves. They taught that we are all sinners and that it is a sin to think highly of yourself. At least that's the message I got.

It seems they taught me that I was worthless. It resonated because it's what I already believed. *I am worthless*, I thought. It would take another 10 years to understand how limiting that belief was.

And I gradually began the process of unraveling my limiting beliefs about God; who God is, what God wants, why God created me, who I am, and why that's important.

How my checkbook changed my attitude

I discovered that my beliefs were not necessarily facts and that some of them were stopping me. Years later, I finally discovered that it's me who decides whether or not to "like" something and that deciding to like it, or at least not hate it, changes everything. First I decided to "like" balancing my checkbook and controlling my household money rather than hating finances and letting them control me. That led to learning to want to make my bed and do the dishes, instead of not wanting to do those things. And that led to wanting to test my blood sugar.

See, I changed my first limiting beliefs simply by deciding that what I believed wasn't serving my higher good. My limiting beliefs were hindering my progress by making it hard. After all, if you don't want to keep track of your expenditures how easy will it be to keep control of your money?

Start by identifying one limiting belief that's hurting you. If you have trouble, refer to my list of limiting beliefs in Chapter 8 and start with something from that list.

Step 6 Challenge and change your limiting beliefs

Now it's much easier and quicker to change my limiting beliefs. All I have to do is identify a belief that is not serving me and I am able to change it. Recently I changed a belief that I don't like the field of sales. I never considered myself a sales person but in truth many things we do in life are *sales* by nature. If I don't embrace sales how do you think I'll do at writing and selling the truths in this book? And since they are truths it will be important to sell them – that is, to get the message across to the people who need to hear it. Selling is nothing more than figuring out to whom to deliver the message and how to get the message to them in a way that they will receive.

So I simply decided I *am* in sales and I proceeded from that thinking to the things you have seen in this book. Instead of hiding from selling or running from it I embraced it. That's the most organic way to change a belief. Changing a belief is harder when it's a belief that goes against the grain. So when it's not a characteristic of my personality and yet needs changing, I will do a Psych-K® balance to change it.

The beliefs in my table (Chapter 8) reflect the ones I used Psych-K® balancing to change. Anything outside your personality, that is thoughts or ideas uncharacteristic of you, are not at the core of your personality and are much harder to change. Nevertheless, they can be changed and I change mine when they are getting in my way.

Step 7 Write your authentic diabetes code

Here is a complete list of all the tools I have given you to create your code.

To begin, complete *Worksheet 1. Complete Worksheet 2* every day for at least a week.

Step 1. What you experienced when you were diagnosed.
- Tell the story of the experiences that led to your diagnosis.
- What did you feel?
- What did you think about?

Step 2. List all the things that are not right in your life.
- Make a complete list.
- Add to it as you identify others.
- Complete the *Current Problem* and *Your Current Code* columns of the worksheet *Your Diabetes Code.*

Step 3. Identify the problem at the core. Don't stop until you hit on the core issue.

Step 4. Begin work to heal the core DIS-ease
- Work on everything on your list but focus most importantly on that one core problem you identified.
- Begin to do things you have not been doing.
- Begin to do things differently than you have been doing them.

Step 5. Identify your limiting beliefs one by one
- Identify one limiting belief that's hurting you.
- If you have trouble, start with something from my list.
- Complete the *Old Belief* column of the Belief Change Worksheet.

Step 6. Challenge and change your limiting beliefs one at a time

- No belief is a fact.
- Some of the most limiting beliefs are religious ones.
- If you realize that a task you must do is limiting you because you don't like it, decide what there is *to like* about it, or why you believe it's not *likeable*.

Step 7. Write your Authentic Diabetes Code. Include codes for all four areas (from Chapter 1).

1. Practical: Actions you want to take including information from your health care providers, and the tools and diet practices you want to adopt. Pump, meter, dosage calculator, carbohydrate tables, etc.

2. Mental: Knowledge about diabetes, diabetes management, online forums, periodicals and books. Learning more and better ways, including changes in your diet, how you feel about your health care providers, what you like about your current system, and what you don't like about it.

3. Emotional: How you deal with anger, resentment, guilt, fear, and apathy. How joy, love, and forgiveness will factor in.

4. Spiritual: Beliefs about God, other people, yourself, your body, and your life.

5. Soulful: Activities you love to do, objects you love to look at and touch, environments you love to be in, foods you love to eat, everything you enjoy with your senses, people you love to be with, and your pets.

Use this entire chapter and the following worksheets and tables:
Worksheet 1
Worksheet 2
Belief Change Worksheet

Step 8 Support your new code every day

Once your code is written make one condensed version, a simple list, and post it in a prominent place. Before long you will know your new code by heart, the same as you did your old one, and you will automatically practice it, like I do mine.

When I first began this process I thought that I could not change an action and sustain it without first changing the underlying belief. I have since learned that's not exactly true. Your new actions will help change your attitudes. It's the new action that reinforces the change in your beliefs.

I sustain my commitment to a healthy body by following my own advice. When I read my own advice I do better. When I fall into old habits I can always identify that I have not been reading my own book. Let this book inspire you to take care of yourself, just as it inspires me.

When you want to form a new belief, don't just try to change the belief – begin by changing some of the behaviors you do that support the old belief. When you have made a new action into a habit it will probably surprise you that a core belief has changed. New beliefs can help you change your actions *and* new actions can also help to change your beliefs. That's how affirmations work (Chapter 8). New actions are a way you can support your new diabetes code every day.

Important Aspects of My Code

Physical/Practical: Actions I wanted to take, including information from my health care providers and deciding for myself what I thought of the care my health care providers were providing.

- Began seeing a Naturopathic doctor who helps me understand my body in ways my traditional doctors never have.

- Investigated diet practices which included learning more about nutrition, other than what the typical dietitian teaches.
- Researched and purchased the single best investment I have ever made – a diabetes dosage calculator in an iPhone app called RapidCalc that only cost $6 and took a big part of the trouble and the sting out of diabetes control.
- Investigated tools I wanted to adopt; insulin pump, meters, dosage calculators, carbohydrate tables, and other inventions to make my life easier.
- Regular attendance at my local annual Diabetes Expo.
- Regular exercise which includes taking my dogs on long walks.

Soulful: Ways to think and actions to take to care deeply about myself. Activities I love to do, objects I love to look at and touch, environments I love to be in, foods I love to eat, everything I enjoy with my senses, people I love to be with, travel, and my pets.

- Writing this book, which has inspired me so much. I love to read it and reread it, and when I do it has the power to make me take responsibility. Writing and rereading this book teaches me so much and my *labor of love* is for myself as well as for you.
- The people in my life who love and support me. My husband, siblings, friends, and co-workers. And even strangers.
- Giving back, paying it forward, and becoming more interdependent. We all need people and people need us. The more loving I am the more love I experience.
- My four adorable miniature dachshunds who love me unconditionally, whom I love unconditionally, and who teach me the definition of true love.
- My love of cooking and inventing creations in the kitchen that are both delicious and healthy.
- Knitting, through which I connect with my mother who taught me. I feel her near me whenever I knit, even though she died in

1975. Knitting connects me with my daughter who loves to knit and who lives 1000 miles away.

- Gardening which connects me to earth, ground, and roots.

Mental: Knowledge about diabetes; diabetes management, online forums, periodicals and books. Learning more and better ways, including what I like and what I don't like about the system I use to care for myself.

- I purchased books to further my diabetes research (see the resource section) such as *The 50 Secrets of the Longest Living People with Diabetes* and *Primal Body, Primal Mind*.
- I joined online diabetes forums like Diabetic Connect at http://www.diabeticconnect.com.
- I researched websites for current updates on diabetes
    - o American Diabetes Association
      http://www.diabetes.org
    - o American Association of Diabetes Educators
      www.diabeteseducator.org
    - o http://www.whyinsulin.com; and the National Diabetes Information clearing house at
      www.diabetes.niddk.nih.gov

Emotional: How I deal with anger, resentment, guilt, fear, and apathy. How I can have more joy and love.

- I can decide whether I want to like or dislike anything. I decided not to hate having diabetes.
- I do not want to live with chronic low-level emotions so I learned to simply let them go.
- I go *through* emotions rather than trying to avoid them or self-medicate.
- I use tools like the ones found in Chapter 8 to release emotions and turn around low energy.

- I forgive, knowing it does not need to be threatening; it is a form of self-love; it is an emotional release that allows me to be happier and more loving.
- I understand that anger, frustration, and fear are natural and I will have these feelings. But that doesn't mean they control me.

Spiritual: Beliefs about God, other people, myself, my body, and my life.

- My beliefs are what I decide they are. No one tells me what to believe. My high-self guides me in what I believe.
- I have learned to recognize beliefs that no longer serve me and to use a specially designed process to literally change them to beliefs that support who I am.
- I listen to my higher power and try my best to not let the 3-year-old (my ego) be in charge of me.

Chapter 11. Your new Code: Putting it All Together

I like my little hand. I haven't always liked it. And it hasn't always been easy. But it has taught me an important lesson: that life isn't easy and it isn't always fair. But if we can make the most out of what we've been given, and find our own way of doing things, you wouldn't believe what can happen.

~ Jim Abbott, Major League Baseball pitcher,
born with no right hand

Get connected to your higher power

When you are connected to your higher power nothing is impossible. You have it within you to make this journey. No one said it will be easy, in fact it's difficult. Few will even begin to make the effort, or continue to make it when it becomes even more difficult. Remember, the hardest part of a journey is the first step. You have all the available people, resources, and tools to help you get started and to continue to help you when it gets tough.

Get to Know You

What do Cark Jung, Abraham Maslow, Joseph Campbell, Albert Einstein, and the Buddha have in common? Their message was the same; life is about knowing who you are. The greatest journey you can make is the one you make inside yourself. When you are certain of who you are there is no limit to what's possible. It's not an easy journey though. It's *The Road Not* [usually] *Taken* (Robert Frost).

Your most valuable resource is you. Have you ever accomplished something incredible? Where did the strength, knowledge, and perseverance come from? They are all part of your amazing package. You have a body and mind capable of the actions needed to accomplish what you may have considered improbable, impossible, or even downright fool hardy.

When a goal feels impossible, consult your inner-most guide; you have an inner knowing-ness that transcends all that your logic seems to say. It will be your job to stay focused on that higher knowledge and to remember you can do it! The more you accomplish the better you will be at trusting your inner guide.

Find Your Community and Stay Connected

When the goal becomes hard there is always someone or some group that can support you. Find your community – that you feel connected with, where the people understand and support you, and where they accept you for exactly who you are. This can be a group of people who share your illness, a church group, a social group, or whatever group works for you.

But stay connected with people. Be open to them – talk about what you are going through. Don't be afraid or ashamed to admit your fears, your doubts, and your anger. The help you get may surprise you.

Change Your New Actions into Habits

A pregnancy takes nine months. My pregnancy with my daughter, when I was new to Type 1 diabetes, seemed too difficult at times. I had to stay on an extremely rigid diet, stay away from simple carbs, monitor my blood sugar constantly, call my nurse daily to report my results, visit my doctor every two weeks, and worry that all my effort was not going to be good enough. I was overjoyed when at three months the tests confirmed a normal, healthy fetus. But my true reward came when my daughter was born healthy and normal, without any of the complications we had worried about. And all I could think of at that point was to love and care for my precious baby girl. Gone was the worry, gone was the frustration, and gone was the difficulty of managing a high risk pregnancy.

The success of developing your authentic diabetes code and actualizing the life of your dreams is like that. At the beginning of this book we discussed habits; it takes 21 days to form a new neural pathway in your brain to support any new habit. I recommend working on one goal at a time. That's why I keep saying all this takes time. People give up because they are overwhelmed looking at all the work it is going to take, and because they don't see enough progress. So don't look at all the work. Look only at what you are currently working on.

Where I live I get to look across the valley at a large mountain called Lone Peak. It's about six miles away. It's an amazing mountain and when I work from my home I look out at it from my office window. If I wanted to walk to that mountain and back it would take me an entire day. Suppose I started walking toward it. If there were nothing between my house and the mountain I would probably go about a mile and it might not seem to me that I was any closer; it would still look just as far away. By that time I would probably start feeling impatient.

It would only be by looking back and seeing my house, small now back in the distance that I would be able to see how truly far I had come. It would make me feel less overwhelmed and I would gain energy from looking back at the distance I had traveled. That achievement would motivate me to continue on. The way to measure your progress is by looking back.

When you feel overwhelmed by the size of your goal, just look back at where you were when you began. Look at the beginning, look back to the time a few months previous when you began to make a few changes, and then look again at a significant breakthrough you made. Keeping track of your milestones will give you an exact moment to look back upon and remember how it felt. Then you can renew the promise you made to yourself.

People give up before they even begin to see significant change. But change is slowest at the very beginning, before the change gains momentum. That's why people give up. That's where my experience and the stories of others will help. Listen to me and others who have been on similar journeys. Talk with them. Read about them. Believe them. And be willing to be patient with yourself.

Believe me when I tell you that when you are in the habit of living according to your code, when you have changed your thoughts, beliefs, and behaviors, you will not remember how difficult it was to get started. It will be like me, when I looked into the eyes of my healthy, whole, adorable baby girl. You will hardly remember that it was ever difficult.

It will be like being in orbit, taking only small amounts of fuel to stay on track. In three months you will notice an immense difference. In a year you will automatically monitor, correct, and go on with the life you want as you are creating it to be. And the journey will not be over, it will be just beginning.

When you think about diabetes it will be no big thing; just a bump in the road of a happy life. You will test, manage, and report your progress because it's no big deal, and because it has become effortless. When you want to do more, subscribe to diabetes magazines, join an online forum, adjust your diet, and try new recipes. Continue as I do to add new things to your code as you come up with them. Who knows? You may heal completely and not even have the physical symptoms of diabetes. If you still have the symptoms you will have no trouble managing them and living a full life. You will have all the energy you need to be a healthy and happy person with or without diabetes.

Conclusion

Do you not see how necessary a world of pains and troubles is to school an intelligence and make it a soul?

~John Keates

Carefully consider every aspect of your disease. We do so much without thinking. There are so many things to hate about life – so many things to hate about diabetes. But hating anything makes it that much harder to manage. Liking or hating something is a decision you decide to make. You will need to decide to feel differently about diabetes and to change your approach if you want to make managing it easier.

How much does diabetes seem to take away from living the life you want?

What gets in your way? Is it managing your diet, your emotions, your low energy or troubling relationships? Are you without health insurance? Do you feel overwhelmed and do you shut down when you think about trying to change any of the things that are getting in your way?

Start with one thing then. Don't try to tackle it all at once. Remember – one bite at a time.

List the things you need to do and create a plan for each one. Then take them on individually. Start with one item and make your solution significant. Plan, implement, adjust, practice, monitor your progress, and track your milestones. And remember to celebrate your progress as you go and to look back on where you were to gain perspective.

Push through the hard part and it will get easier. I promise you it will become downright effortless. Your blueprint is based on *your* idea of control, not someone else's. Your inner coach will help you come up with your plan.

Put the education into action by living your plan every day, even while it is in its unfinished state. Let it change and develop as you change and develop. Think about the bigger picture. What are you here to accomplish? What have you always loved doing? What have you stopped pursuing because you have symptoms of a disease?

It's not hard to become happy and healthy with diabetes; if I did it anyone can. You've read my stories so you know that it's true. I've shared my stories so that people everywhere will see the possibilities for their lives. I hope you surpass my success and exceed any expectations you have had for your own life.

And remember that you are here at the *school of life* to live the life of your dreams. You are not here to hide in the shadow of any disease.

Appendix A. The Best Alkaline Foods for pH Balance

Basic pH Content of Common Foods

Neutral/Mildly Alkaline-producing Foods: vegetables, fruits, organic grains, nuts	Better Acid-producing Foods: fruits, some grains and fats, foods high but lower in acidity	Highly Acidic Foods: Meat, poultry, grains, nuts, refined foods, sweets, fats, beverages
Almonds	Acai Berries	Alcohol
Almond Milk	Apples	Artificial sweeteners
Apples	Bananas	Beef
Asparagus	Barley	Beer
Avocado	Black Beans	Beet sugar
Beans	Brown /Basmati Rice	Brown Rice Syrup
Bee Pollen	Butter	Candy
Beets	Blueberries	Canned Fruit and Vegetables
Bell Peppers	Brown rice syrup	Cheese (hard)
Borage Oil	Buffalo	Chicken
Bottled Water: Fiji, Evian, Hawaiian	Cantaloupe	Chocolate
Brazil nuts	Cashews	Cocoa
Broccoli	Cherries	Coffee

(Neutral/Mildly Alkaline-producing)	(Better Acid-producing Foods)	(Highly Acidic Foods)
Brussels sprouts	Chicken	Deli Meat
Buckwheat	Coconut Milk	Deep Fried Foods
Buttermilk	Cooked/frozen vegetables	Dried Fruit
Cabbage	Cod Liver Oil	Eggs
Carrots	Corn	Fish (Farmed)
Cauliflower	Cream	Fruit Juice
Coconut (fresh)	Dates	Jam/Jelly
Cucumber	Fish (wild caught)	Ketchup
Fish Oil	Fresh water fist	Liquor
Flax seeds	Fruit juice	Mayonnaise
Garlic	Grapefruit	Miso
Horseradish	Grapeseed Oil	Molasses
Lemon	Hazelnuts	Mushrooms
Lettuce	Honey	Mustard
Limes	Hummus	Pickles
Mushrooms	Macadamia nuts	Pineapple
Navy Beans	Margarine	Pork
Olive Oil	Milk (homogenized)	Sardines
Onions	Oatmeal	Shellfish
Peas (fresh)	Organ meats	Soda pop
Pine Nuts (raw)	Oysters	Soy sauce
Potatoes	Peaches, pears	Syrup
Quinoa	Peanuts	Tea (Black)
Raw Honey	Raspberries	Tuna (canned)
Seaweed	Raw Milk	Veal
Sesame Oil	Rice Milk	Vinegar
Soy Beans	Rye bread	Wine
Soy flour	Strawberries	Yeast
Spinach	Sweet Potatoes	

(Neutral/Mildly Alkaline-producing)	(Better Acid-producing Foods)	(Highly Acidic Foods)
Sprouts	Tea (Green)	
Summer squash	Turbinado sugar	
Sunflower seeds	Whey Protein Powder	
Sweet potatoes	Whole grain bread	
Tomatoes	Whole grain pasta	
Yams	Whole meal bread	
Zucchini	Winter Squash	

Source: http://www.alkalinesisters.com/alkaline-food-chart/

Appendix B. A Return to the Basics: the Paleo Diet

The ideas considered here contradict the advice given by most medical professionals today, as well as opposing those of general medical science, the US government, and even the majority of the modern general population. They have saved many lives whereas the orthodox theories our current nutritional system subscribes to only seem to be exacerbating the problems of modern health – our *diseases of civilization*. This is a brief overview of some ideas that seek to bring our species back into harmony with nature.

For most of our evolution the world has been a very different place than the one we live in today. Recent analysis of primitive diets concludes that animal-source foods and fat-soluble nutrients played a critical role in the remarkable physical and mental health as well as in the freedom from disease that is characteristic of primitive, Paleolithic peoples. In fact, our ice age physiology has evolved little adaptation to, or defense against, carbohydrates.

Diets high in carbohydrates are a modern phenomenon. In fact, of all the macronutrients (protein, fat, and carbohydrate) the only one for which there is no actual human dietary requirement is carbohydrate. This is critical; *we don't have to eat starch of any kind in order to be optimally healthy.*

"Excess consumption of sugar, starch, and cereal-based carbohydrates is easily the most destructive dietary tendency today. It is a rampant problem, leading to heart disease, obesity, diabetes, cancer, and many other degenerative disorders as well as numerous mental health and cognitive problems."

~Nora T. Gedgaudas, CNS, CNT
Author of *Primal Body, Primal Mind*

Insulin resistance, known in the medical world as Syndrome X, is associated with unusually high consumption of omega-6 fats (vegetable oils) and, to a lesser degree, omega-9 fats (olive and oleic oils). Low-fat diets have not prevented heart disease, which is increasing; obesity, which affects approximately 58 percent of the US population; diabetes, the most common result of insulin resistance and recognized to have reached epidemic proportions; or cancer, now the leading cause of death in the US.

Conversely, DHA, an essential omega-3 fatty acid, makes up the highest percentage of fat in the human brain. Omega-3 acids are found in grass-fed products (milk, eggs, butter, meat fat, and organs), and in wild-caught cold-water fish.

Compare the healthy lives and bodies of our pre-agricultural Paleolithic ancestors with modern Homo sapiens. The decline in stature, bone density, and dental health, together with the increases in birth defects, malnutrition, and disease, which have followed the wide-spread implementation of farming and an increased intake of grains, shows the extreme digression since modern man left behind the naturally high-fat, moderate-protein, hunter-gatherer diets we are genetically programmed for.

Our farming-based, grain based, carbohydrate-rich lifestyle, according to Gedgaudas, as well as many more naturopathic physicians and nurse practitioners, has led to lifelong weight gain, cravings, mood disorders, and the diseases of civilization – cancer, osteoporosis, insulin resistance, heart disease, diabetes, and mental illness.

The information certainly makes a case for a return to mankind's original Paleo diet.

Related Reading

Your "Healthy" Diet Could Be Quietly Killing Your Brain. *Grain Brain*, by Dr. David Perlmutter challenges convention with the latest science on brain health. As discussed in Psychology Today. https://www.psychologytoday.com/blog/the-optimalist/201310/your-healthy-diet-could-be-quietly-killing-your-brain published by Max Lugavere on Oct 09, 2013 in The Optimalist retrieved May 20, 2015.

Obesity Itself Not a Diabetes Risk by Cole Petrochko, MedPage Today, Sept 18, 2012. Article.
http://www.medpagetoday.com/PrimaryCare/Obesity/34819.

Appendix C. Basic Muscle Testing Instructions

Muscle movements, our motor functions, are directed by the subconscious part of the mind. Thus, Muscle testing is a built-in communication link to the subconscious mind. George Goodheart, D.C., the founder of Applied Kinesiology, introduced muscle testing in the United States more than thirty years ago. It is effective in communicating with the conscious mind the beliefs we hold on to that limit our ability to live full lives and to be all we are capable of being (Williams, 2009).

During the thought process the signal strength to your muscles increases or decreases depending on the feeling a thought produces. A reduction in the electrical signal from the brain reduces the strength of the muscle and causes a weak response. It's a binary code of simple *yes* or *no* answers that you can read yourself. The significance of this is you may think you believe one way when in reality *your body energy is telling you that you believe something surprisingly different or even the opposite of what you thought.*

Once you understand muscle testing and can identify your own muscle responses, you can begin to experiment on muscles like your legs and your fingers. Until then you will want to use a partner and test the deltoid muscle in your arm.

Determine which arm to use. It can be either arm unless one arm is sore or injured. Stand facing your partner slightly to the side and looking at the shoulder of the arm you are going to test.

Have your partner extend his arm out to the side so it is parallel to the floor. Keep one hand resting lightly on the extended arm between the wrist and the elbow and place your other hand on his shoulder to give you stability.

Have your partner keep his body relaxed and his head facing forward, and have him focus on the floor at a point about four feet out in front of him. Have him keep his chin parallel to the floor and just point his eyes down.

Have him think of something he likes. It can be a person, activity, thing, or place. Thinking of foods you enjoy works very well. When your partner is experiencing the good feeling say, "Be strong" and apply gentle but steady pressure on the arm downward for about two seconds or until you feel the muscle either "let go" or "lock in place." Do not bounce or apply hard pressure. Your partner is to resist your pressure while thinking the enjoyable thought.

- Note whether the response was strong or weak.
- Trade places and have your partner do the test on you.

Next, tell your partner to imagine something unpleasant and repeat the process, giving him enough time to experience the feeling of it before applying pressure. Notice any difference between the pleasant and the unpleasant thought and feeling. Most people test strong to the pleasant thought (the arm stays parallel to the floor) and weak to the unpleasant one (the arm moves down toward the floor even as the person tries to keep it parallel). The person being tested must be able to tell the difference for the test to be considered successful.

To ensure the test will be accurate on a critical life issue test several times holding different thoughts. Try saying "My name is _____" your real name, and then again with a name that is not yours. Then try repeating "yes, yes, yes" to yourself, then "no, no, no." You will be pleasantly surprised!

Notes about muscle testing:

You can alternate between arms if the one you are working with gets tired, since the test works on either arm. Everyone tests differently so you will need different amounts of pressure to suit each person. You only need to press as hard and as long as necessary in order for you and your partner to tell whether the response is strong or weak. It's good to ask questions as you go.

The most important point is to understand whether the person being tested can tell whether the test was strong or weak. Keeping the face forward and eyes down and outward about four feet accesses the necessary part of the brain to give an accurate result.

Remember to say the words, "Be strong" each time before applying pressure.

If a test gives you erratic responses it could be a neurological disorder of some type. More often the person being tested just needs water.

A degree of skepticism is normal but unless the person being tested is open to the process they can skew their own results. Make sure all parties are in agreement before attempting to test.

Most people I have personally muscle tested achieve normal results. I have only seen a few skewed results, once due to metal plates and screws in the shoulder and a few times due to an unwillingness to "play" on the part of the person being tested. To guard against this I always ask permission before entering someone's personal space. I ask if it's OK if I stand here, if I touch their arm, etc. It helps prepare the other person to allow you to conduct the test. But do not rely too heavily on your own results of muscle testing. There are a number of reasons your results may be skewed.

Quotes and Citations

P 9   Butler, David. From a private conversation circa 1989

P 23   Aristotle

P 54   Albert Einstein. (n.d.).,

P 83   William Shakespeare

P 129 Bud Light Journey Commercial Stevie Wonder February 2013

P 129 Alexandra Asseily, from the film *The Power of Forgiveness* by Martin Doblmeier. 2008. https://www.journeyfilms.com/?s=the+poser+of+forgiveness

P 131 Dwoskin, H. 2003. *The Sedona Method: Your Key to Lasting Happiness, Success, Peace, and Emotional Well-Being.* Sedona Press, Sedona AZ www.sedona.com

P 138 Williams, R. 2009. *PSYCH-K®: The Missing* ~~Piece~~ *Peace in Your Life.* Myrddin Corp, CO. www.psych-k.com

P 145 Carrington, P. PhD. 2008. *Discover the Power of Meridian Tapping.* The Tapping Solution, LLC, Newtown, CT

P 150 Gunderson, G. 2009. *Freedom Fasttrack* Seminar, Salt Lake City, UT

P 155 Sanskrit Proverb from the Mahakavi Kalidasa

P 179 Jim Abbott. From Abbott, J and T. Brown. 2012. *Imperfect: an Improbable Life.* Random House, New York, NY

Referenced Works

P 9   Common Symptoms of Stress compiled from personal notes and general information on symptoms of stress and anxiety, including the DSM IV (Diagnostic and Statistical Manual of Mental Disorders, 4th Edition).

P 28   Reprinted with the permission of Scribner, a Division of Simon & Schuster, Inc., from THE PEOPLE CODE: IT'S ALL ABOUT YOUR INNATE MOTIVE by Dr. Taylor Hartman. Copyright © 1997 by Taylor Hartman. All rights reserved.

P 46   Loehr, J. and T. Schwartz. 2003. *The Power of Full Engagement.* Simon & Schuster, Inc. New York, NY

P 62   Canfield, J. *The Success Principles: How to Get from Where You Are to Where You Want to Be.* 2005. HarperCollins, New York, NY

P 69   *Maximum Confidence* CD program, Jack Canfield 2002. Nightingale-Conant, Simon & Schuster Audio

P 74   Lipton, B. 2005. *The Biology of Belief.* Hay House, New York, NY

P 76   Gedgaudas, N. CNS, CNT. 2011. *Primal Body, Primal Mind .* Inner Traditions International and Bear & Company. All rights reserved. http://www.Innertraditions.com

P 78   Alkaline Sisters. Visit http://www.alkalinesisters.com

P 97   Mallinger, A. and J. DeWyze. 1992. *Too Perfect: When Being in Control Gets Out of Control.* Random House, New York, NY

P 106   Dwoskin, H. 2003. *The Sedona Method: Your Key to Lasting Happiness, Success, Peace, and Emotional Well-Being.* Sedona Press, Sedona AZ www.sedona.com

P 115   Hill, N. 1937. *Think and Grow Rich.* The Napoleon Hill Foundation, Hammond, IN

P 126   Abbott, J. and T. Brown. 2012. *Imperfect: an Improbable Life*. Random House, New York, NY

P 169 *Maximum Confidence* CD program, Jack Canfield 2002. Nightingale-Conant, Simon & Schuster Audio

P 172   Williams, R. 2009. *PSYCH-K®: The Missing ~~Piece~~ Peace in Your Life*. Myrddin Corp, CO. www.psych-k.com

P 175   RapidCalc Insulin dose iPhone app – The Apple App Store

P 180   Frost, R. "The Road Not Taken." *Selected Poems of Robert Frost*. 1963. New York: Holt, Rinehart and Winston. New York, NY.

P 189   Alkaline Sisters. Visit http://www.alkalinesisters.com/alkaline-food-chart/. Retrieved Mar 17, 2016

Resources

Articles

The Relationship of Sugar to Population-Level Diabetes Prevalence: An Econometric Analysis of Repeated Cross-Sectional Data *by Sanjay Basu, Paula Yoffe, Nancy Hills, Robert H. Lustig*, PloS One, Feb 27, 2013. Available at
http://www.plosone.org/article/info%3Adoi%2F10.1371%2Fjournal.pone.0057873

Related:
It's the Sugar, Folks *by Mark Bittman*. NY Times Opinion Pages Feb 27, 2013
http://opinionator.blogs.nytimes.com/2013/02/27/its-the-sugar-folks/

Depression: Your Brain on Sugar by Sarah the Healthy Home Economist, Feb 7, 2012 available at
http://www.thehealthyhomeeconomist.com/depression-your-brain-on-sugar/

8 Foods You Should Eat Every Day, Men's Health June 20, 2009 available at http://www.menshealth.com/nutrition/superfoods-for-men

10 Psychosocial problems and barriers to improved diabetes management results of the Cross-National Diabetes Attitudes, Wishes and Needs (DAWN) Study Nov 11, 2004 available at http://www.dawnyouth.com/documents/dawn%20materials/dawn_publications/10_psychosocial_problems_and_barriers.pdf

Depression and Poor Glycemic Control Diabetes Care Volume 23 Number 7 July 2000 available at http://care.diabetesjournals.org/content/23/7/934.

Diabetes websites:

- American Diabetes Association http://www.diabetes.org/
- American Association of Diabetes Educators www.diabeteseducator.org
- ADA American Dietetic Association www.eatright.org
- AACE American Association of Clinical Endocrinologists www.aace.com
- CDE a healthcare professional certified in diabetes education - www.CDEhelpteam.com
- National diabetes information clearing house www.diabetes.niddk.nih.gov

Support from the Diabetes Community:

- Diabetic Connect http://www.diabeticconnect.com
- DLife http://dlife.com
- Diabetes Sisters. https://www.diabetessisters.org/

Recommended Reading

Be Your Own Shaman: Heal Yourself and Others with 21st-Century Energy Medicine, by Deborah King. 2011. Hay House, New York, NY. This book will help you find the power to heal yourself. King uses centuries-old Eastern and Western practices from up to 5000 years ago, combined with modern concepts to form a cutting-edge approach to health and healing. This book will open you up to power you never knew you had and give you the confidence to tap into it.

The Biology of Belief: Unleashing the Power of Consciousness, Matter, & Miracles by Bruce H. Lipton, PhD. 2007. Hay House, New York, NY.
The research by Dr. Bruce Lipton will open your eyes to the things you can't see. Dr. Lipton and his colleagues have made amazing discoveries about the interaction between your mind and your body and the processes by which cells receive information. Mainstream science could very possibly be wrong. According to Lipton, genes and DNA do not control our biology. DNA is actually controlled by signals from outside the cell, including the energetic messages emanating from our thoughts. *The Biology of Belief* will change how you think about thinking.

Care of the Soul : A Guide for Cultivating Depth and Sacredness in Everyday Life by Thomas Moore. 1992. Harper Collins, New York, NY.
In one of my all-time favorite books Thomas Moore provides a fresh focus on the idea of soul as well as concrete ways to foster soulfulness in the ordinary living of our lives. Soulfulness deepens and strengthens us, providing in us a heart-centered complexity. Moore borrows heavily from mythology and uses the works of Carl Jung and others like him to

teach us how to take care of our souls. I keep picking up this book again and again. I can't read it enough.

American Diabetes Association Complete Guide to Diabetes: The Ultimate Home Reference from the Diabetes Experts. 2011. The American Diabetes Association.

This is simply the comprehensive home reference for when you need information to manage your diabetes symptoms. The 5th edition volume contains information on self-care techniques and medical advances in diabetes care. Topics include the latest on self-care for type 1, type 2, and gestational diabetes; new types of insulin and medications; strategies for avoiding diabetes complications; expanded sections on meal planning and nutrition (please take some of this information with a grain of salt); and tips on working with the health care system and insurance providers.

Dark Nights of the Soul: A Guide to Finding Your Way through Life's Ordeals, by Thomas Moore. 2005. Penguin Books, New York, NY.

We tend to look at the dark periods in life as obstacles that must be overcome as quickly as possible. This is because we are uncomfortable with their sadness, weakness, and dark emotions. But deep healing cannot be forced to happen quickly. Moore's approach is to dive more deeply into the story of St. John of the Cross to discover the meaning of the darker side of life. He honors life's fragile, vulnerable times and teaches how to create depth and healing not possible with immediate remedies.

Bradshaw On: The Family: A New Way of Creating Solid Self-Esteem by John Bradshaw. 1990. Health Communications, Inc. Deerfield Beach, FL.

This is part of a culmination of Bradshaw's popular 1980's PBS series, when Bradshaw popularized the term *inner child*. Through this timeless wisdom Bradshaw discusses toxic shame, emotionally impaired families, how unhealthy rules of behavior perpetuate in families, and the destructive effect all of this has on our society. This is your go-to book for learning how to create healthy relationships.

50 Secrets of the Longest Living People with Diabetes, by Sheri R. Colberg and Steven V. Edelman. 2007. Marlowe & Company, Cambridge, MA.
The longest living people with type 1 and type 2 diabetes share the secrets that have helped them achieve longevity and wellness, featuring interviews with more than 50 people who have thrived with diabetes for as many as 84 years. You'll be inspired by their stories. It could help *you* live longer too.

The Four Agreements: A Practical Guide to Personal Freedom by Don Miguel Ruiz. 1997. Amber Allen Publishing, San Rafael, CA.
Don Miguel Ruiz possesses powerful insight that reveals both the cause and the cure of self-limiting beliefs that rob us of joy and create needless suffering, based on ancient Toltec wisdom. Don't take anything personally. Be impeccable with your word. Don't make assumptions. Always do your best. This book can transform your life with how and why we should keep these four agreements with ourselves.

Loving What Is: Four Questions That Can Change Your Life, by Byron Katie. Katie, B. 2002. Three Rivers Press, New York, NY.
The Work consists of four questions that can be applied to a specific problem in order to be able to look at what is troubling you from an entirely different perspective. Trying to let go of a painful thought doesn't work. Diving beneath the surface of the problem does. Through The Work people find a more lasting peace, even in times when they had previously thought it was impossible.

Maximum Confidence CD program, by Jack Canfield 2002. Nightingale-Conant, Simon & Schuster Audio.
The very best resource for anyone who wants to restore their self-esteem and gain more confidence. In this program, self-esteem guru Jack

Canfield, with his friendly, personable approach, easily invites you to partake in exercises and perspectives that will increase yourself-esteem whether you aware of it or not.

The People Code: it's All about Your Innate Motive, by Taylor Hartman. 1997. Simon & Schuster, New York, NY.

Unlike most personality profile programs, Hartman takes an approach to personality based on core motivators, which are innate, not learned. It is due to these core motivators, love, joy, power, and peace, that we react to and operate in our various environments, differently than the way other people would, given the same situation. When you understand what motivates you at your very core you are ready to take on the world on your own terms.

The Power of Forgiveness. A film by Martin Doblmeier. 2008. Journey Films. www.journeyfilms.com and www.firstrunfeatures.com.

This film looks at forgiveness on various levels besides what we are taught about forgiveness in Sunday School. It examines the science behind forgiveness. Physical ramifications of not forgiving include heightened anxiety and blood pressure; it shows how having or not having forgiveness affects our health. And it shows the power of forgiveness on a societal level; how our world could be different if forgiveness were taken seriously and widely practiced. This DVD will transform you if you're open to forgiving, and it will help you become open if you're not.

The Power of Full Engagement, by Jim Loehr and Tony Schwartz. 2003. Simon & Schuster, Inc. New York, NY.

This inspired work helped me understand the details behind the idea that *everything is energy* and why and how people waste their precious energy in huge quantities. These sports psychologists examined hours of footage to discover what differentiates top athletes. They discovered that it is in the ways they conserve energy that are counter to the ways their competitors are using it up. We only have a precious, finite amount of energy to motivate us and keep us going. It will be up to you to learn how.

Primal Body, Primal Mind by Nora T. Gedgaudas. CNS, CNT published by Inner Traditions International and Bear & Company, 2011.
See appendix B. Animal-source foods and fat-soluble nutrients played a critical role in the remarkable physical and mental health, and the freedom from disease that characterizes Paleolithic peoples. Our ice age physiology has evolved little adaptation to carbohydrates. This book is the very best resource I have found on the causes and cures for so-called *diseases of civilization*, most of which have been around for less than 100 years. From the domestication of wheat to cell phones, this book is informative and insightful on one hand, and very difficult to read on the other, especially if you are particularly devoted to carbohydrates, among other things.

The Sedona Method: Your Key to Lasting Happiness, Success, Peace, and Emotional Well-Being, by Hale Dwoskin 2003. Sedona Press, Sedona AZ www.sedona.com.
A simple formula for uncovering the lingering, unpleasant feelings that people often carry around, referred to by psychologists as *emotional baggage*. The Sedona Method is so simple people often miss it. It's as simple as *think about it, and then it's gone.* Jack Canfield said of it that before he found it he used to have seminar attendees beat on pillows for an hour. Once he discovered this method it greatly simplified his life and the lives of thousands of his students.

The Success Principles: How to Get from Where You Are to Where You Want to Be, by Jack Canfield, J. 2005. HarperCollins, New York, NY.
64 timeless principles of life to get you from where you are to where you want to be, beginning with the first principle, Take 100 per cent responsibility for your life. No one else can create the life you want for you. Regardless of your circumstances, you decide where your life will take you. Buy this book, read it, and keep it nearby as you encounter

those times in your life when you will want to have principles for how to deal with events with perspective and class.

Too Perfect: When Being in Control Gets Out of Control, by Mallinger, A. and J. DeWyze. 1992. Random House, New York, NY.
Do you recognize a perfectionist inside of you? This resource will help you understand the difference between perfection and excellence and will help you relax while you strive toward excellence and away from perfectionism, accepting that you are a human being, and therefore, imperfect by your very nature.

Truth Heals: What you hide can hurt you, by Deborah King. 2009. Hay House, Inc. www.hayhouse.com.
The truth can change your life. This book is a roadmap for how to acknowledge and express the thoughts and feelings that are often so painful they are shoved deep down inside. Instead you can learn how you can be healed of their damaging effects. Dr. King's brave approach is straightforward and open. It respects the reader. We lie to each other and we lie to ourselves. And when we continue living with untruths it harms us. This book shows people how they can face the truth about their own lives and take responsibility for healing themselves instead of blaming someone or something else, which gets us nowhere.

About the Author

A few years ago I broke through my own coding to find a world I had not known existed. You might say I woke up to what is most important in life. However, it actually began a few years before that when I finally learned I didn't love myself, and learned how to begin to love myself. That love began to grow into not hating my journey – a journey characterized by the debilitating and disempowering disease, diabetes.

I began to change the limiting beliefs that kept me unhappy and unhealthy. Through my experiences I discovered a much easier and more enjoyable way for anyone to decode the programming that causes us to settle, to play small, and to stay sick; a new code that supports the change I want to be in the world. It feels awesome to be free to live my own dream. Visit http://thediabetesdecoder.com to comment and to read more about current topics.

If you find you have difficulty with any aspect of this book, whether it is in understanding it or implementing it, please contact me. Although all you need to know is in the book achieving it can be very overwhelming and we all need help at times. I can help.

I have lived these concepts steadily for the past eight years. It hasn't always been easy and I haven't always done it perfectly. But living them has helped me become the person I want to be. It helps me live much better with diabetes and I want to help any and all people with diabetes who want help do the same.

Email me at diabetesdecoder@gmail.com and have patience. I will contact you.

Blessings to you…

Sheri

Notes

Notes

Notes

Notes

Notes

Notes

Notes

Notes

Notes